HOLISTIC
PARENTING

HOLISTIC PARENTING

Raising Children to a New

Physical, Emotional,

and Spiritual Well-Being

LYNN WIESE SNEYD

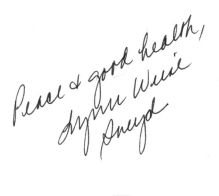

KEATS PUBLISHING

LOS ANGELES

NTC/Contemporary Publishing Group

Library of Congress Cataloging-in-Publication Data

Sneyd, Lynn Wiese.
    Holistic parenting : raising children to a new physical, emotional, and spiritual
well-being / by Lynn Wiese Sneyd.
       p. cm.
    Includes bibiolgraphical references and index.
    ISBN 0-658-00306-2 (paperback)
      1. Pediatrics—Popular works. 2. Children—Diseases—Alternative treatment. 3. Holistic
medicine. I. Title.

RJ61 .S6763 2000
618.92—dc21

00-063438

Published by Keats Publishing
A division of NTC/Contemporary Publishing Group, Inc.
4255 West Touhy Avenue, Lincolnwood, Illinois 60712, U.S.A.

Managing Director and Publisher: Jack Artenstein
Executive Editor: Peter Hoffman
Director of Publishing Services: Rena Copperman
Managing Editor: Jama Carter
Editor: Claudia McCowan
Project Editor: Carmela Carvajal

Text design by Wendy Staroba Loreen

Printed in the United States of America
International Standard Book Number: 0-658-00306-2
00 01 02 03 04 DHD 18 17 16 15 14 13 12 11 10 9 8 7 6 5 4 3 2 1

For Gregg, Hannah, and Elle
My inspiration
My support
My loves

ACKNOWLEDGMENTS

So many wonderful talents, minds, and spirits touched this book. Sheree Bykofsky, my dream agent, adroitly guided it to a most compatible home at Keats Publishing, where it came under the skillful care and editing of Peter Hoffman.

I cannot imagine having completed this project without the support of Debra Brenegan, sister to my writing soul, who spent countless hours reviewing drafts and encouraging me.

Liza Wiemer's extraordinary guidance, shared so patiently and willingly, illuminated much along the winding, dark road.

Most likely, *Holistic Parenting* never would have evolved without the friendship and mentoring of David Russell and his wonderful wife, Tine. In the true tradition of a holistic doctor, David teaches, teaches, teaches, and then teaches some more.

Many other individuals readily shared their time and talents. From beginning to end, Harold Bloomfield, M.D., graciously offered full support. For all their contributions, a thousand heartfelt hugs to Cecil Barton, D.D.S.; Kathleen Long Bostrum; Leslie Bow; Annemarie Colbin; Sue Collins; Pat Coultas; Lee Ann Fagan Dzelzkahns; Judith Fetterly; Jane Friesch; Patricia Hunt; Richard Iammarino, M.D.; Karen Krimmel; Kathy Odenkirk; Mary Reilley; Audrey Ricker, Ph.D.; Diane Rozario; Mary Severin; Mark Sneller, Ph.D.; Gerry Steele; Charles Trimberger, M.S.W.; Stan Posey, L.Ac., Dipl. Ac.; Dana Ullman, M.P.H.; and Marian Wilkerson, R.D. A special thank you to Nancy Wiese and Leslie McIntyre for their editing talents. In addition, I am grateful to the Ragdale Foundation for providing space and solitude.

My parents, who have watched my journey with wonder, concern, and joy but have interfered only with support, sustained me in so many ways.

Without my husband's love, strength, and patience, this book would never have survived beyond its first few tentative steps. His courage and spirit have stood steadfast during challenges far, far more difficult than those encountered during the writing process. I am incredibly proud and thankful to have him beside me.

Finally, this book could not have been written without the two golden-haired angels in my life. They are my mentors and my ballast, the recipients of my parenting errors and successes. And I love them scrumptiously.

I am so richly blessed.

—LYNN WIESE SNEYD
TUCSON, ARIZONA

TABLE OF CONTENTS

FOREWORD

BY HAROLD H. BLOOMFIELD, M.D.

As a medical and psychiatric practitioner, I always keep an eye out for practical resources that I can pass on to patients. I was therefore delighted to discover *Holistic Parenting: Raising Children to a New Physical, Emotional, and Spiritual Well-Being*.

After living through a decade of personal health trials and errors, Lynn Wiese Sneyd decided to explore beyond the boundaries of conventional medicine. During her journey, she discovered that antibiotics are not always necessary for children to heal and immunizations may not be the best prevention against certain diseases. In addition, alternative therapies may treat chronic illness more effectively than conventional medicines. We are so fortunate that this author and mother devoted considerable effort to reviewing the tremendous amount of scientific and medical research presented in this book. If you ever have questioned just how safe and effective homeopathy, herbs, vaccines, genetically engineered food, and fluoride are for your child, then I recommend delving into the following pages.

Laced with humor and lively anecdotes, *Holistic Parenting* does not preach or frighten. It boils down the basics of the holistic, alternative, and integrative medicine movements in a candid, easy-to-read way. The book's style is akin to one parent chatting to another over a backyard fence: "Sammy has a fever, you say? Well, have you ever tried basil tea?" Besides covering the background of alternative therapies and providing scientific data, Wiese Sneyd incorporates suggestions of how to handle the inevitable acute illnesses of childhood—suggestions that might indeed be as basic as opening up your spice and herb cabinet and brewing basil tea to reduce your child's fever.

Speaking as a parent of three children, I extol the simple, inexpensive home care described in this book. Speaking as a Yale-trained physician and psychiatrist, I concur with the author that such safe and effective home care integrates well with professional care, just as Ayurveda, herbal medicine, and homeopathy integrate well with modern medicine.

Crafted with wisdom and love, *Holistic Parenting* is a marvelous resource you will turn to often. After reading it, you will find yourself making simple changes in your lifestyle, diet, and home, not only because it is easy and logical to do so, but also because it profoundly benefits your child. Without a doubt, this book will assist you in the awesome, complex, and rewarding task of child rearing. *Holistic Parenting* is an important and valuable gift for parents and, most of all, their children.

INTRODUCTION

On a frosty January afternoon in 1995, I purged our medicine cabinet. Out went over-the-counter decongestants and digestive aids, pain relievers, and expired prescriptions. After nine years of hair-pulling health challenges, I had learned to use herbs, spices, and foods to help heal the acute illnesses that periodically dampened our spirits. I was finally ready to ordain the kitchen as the family medicine cabinet.

What a journey it had been to that point. When my husband's mysterious illness in 1986 yanked us away from familiar territory, I never suspected that we would drift so far from conventional medicine. Although we weren't yet parents, I always had envisioned being a caring and competent mom who carted kids to the pediatrician for the required shots and picked up prescriptions when some acute malady landed a feverish child under the quilts. Who would have thought a little tingling in the fingertips could initiate such sweeping change?

That's how my husband, Gregg, then aged twenty-seven, described his first symptom back in 1986, when we still lived in Wisconsin. Three years of marriage was enough time to figure out that of the two of us, I was the hypochondriac, ready to diagnose a brain tumor or stroke before a physician even had a chance to lift a stethoscope. So I was surprised and a bit disconcerted when Gregg, the greatest proponent of the maxim "Time will heal," consulted a doctor.

The first nerve conduction studies indicated that something was amiss, that Gregg's nerves were functioning at less than full capacity.

That three-hour test set in motion an arduous diagnostic process that sent us down many a neurology corridor. Spinal taps, MRIs, visits to the Mayo Clinic, a nerve biopsy—Gregg tried every one of them, sometimes repeatedly. All in all, we shook hands with nine neurologists.

The process was enough to cause nerve damage of the mental sort. First, we would schedule a test, usually two weeks down the road. After the test, we'd hold our breaths for another week, waiting for the results, only to learn that more tests were needed. All we could do was eat our bagels in the morning, go to work, and flip our Day-Timer pages as each day dragged by. After eighteen months, the doctors made a diagnosis of a demyelinating asymmetrical peripheral neuropathy, a type of nerve degeneration for which there is no known cause or cure.

"Come back if it gets worse," said one doc.

We stayed away for two years.

During this time, Gregg continued to work and live a normal life on the surface. His nerves, however, no longer moved muscles efficiently, resulting in muscle atrophy and increasing weakness. He slowly lost weight and his hands began to curl involuntarily. A die-hard sports enthusiast, he was forced to take early retirement from intramural basketball and softball. When I saw his glove gathering dust on the basement shelf, I remembered how his once healthy hands nimbly snapped that leather around a ball. Buttoning his shirt collars became part of my morning routine; a persistent weight in the pit of my stomach became part of my life.

Then the choking incidents started. The first time that Gregg's deep, panicked gasps left both of us breathless, a piece of meat, which he would manage to swallow before the paramedics left the station, lodged in his throat. Another time, he choked after gulping water from a bottle during a bike ride. More than once, desperate wheezing pierced my dreams and shoved me into the nightmare of reality. On those dark mornings, my heart raced wildly as I scrambled for the phone, ready to dial 911. It didn't take a diagnostic test or even a doctor to tell me that Gregg's throat muscles were losing strength. We now had a one-year-old, and I couldn't quite swallow the thought of becoming a single parent.

Not seeing any other recourse, we decided to return to the corridors of Western medicine. One neurologist recommended plasmapheresis, a three-hour procedure in which blood is removed through an IV in one arm, cleansed, and returned through an IV in the other arm. The procedure didn't come with guarantees, though insurance did cover its cost, then three thousand dollars. Gregg endured over fifty blood washes over a two-year period. He always drove himself to the hospital, and with bandaged arms, religiously returned to work. When I obtained his medical records, some years later, I was amazed to read the nurse's repeated notes: "Urged patient to have a driver. Patient declined."

Though plasmapheresis seemed to temporarily slow the nerve degeneration, the results were difficult to discern because for the first time since the illness began, the doctor prescribed medicines. Some studies had shown that prednisone—a steroid—and cytoxin—an anticancer drug—might effectively slow degenerative nerve conditions. Within three weeks, this drug cocktail blew Gregg's white blood cell count off the chart and induced diabetes. The doctor had mentioned there was a slight chance this might happen, but not knowing what else to do, we decided to take the risk.

Gregg was still adjusting to using a glucose monitor when he came home early from work one night, frightened. His vision was blurred and he could feel an alarming pressure on the side of his head. He slumped on the couch with his head in his hands, on the verge of tears, wondering how much more he could take. I wasn't sure about my limit either, but it wasn't the time to surmise or mope. My immediate concern was that my husband was about to have a fatal aneurysm. I mentally whizzed through our options. He wasn't at the 911 stage yet. The walk-in clinic was ten minutes away, the emergency room fifteen minutes. I packed up our eighteen-month-old daughter, steered Gregg to the door, and proceeded to break speed limits. The attending physician at the clinic assured us there was no need to operate. He mumbled something about "myasthenia gravis" and prescribed a visit to the neurologist in the morning.

The next day, while waiting for the doctor, I picked up a pamphlet about this myasthenia gravis, a condition in which the nerves stop communicating with the muscles. The pamphlet included a story about a man who got stuck in his bathtub due to one of these communication gaps. I tossed it down, wondering if I should take up weight lifting.

As the pamphlet hit the table, an odd thing happened. It was as if a switch flipped in my mind and a spotlight suddenly illuminated the dark and consuming fear that had rendered us passive in the healing process. For six years, we had responded to doctors with an up-and-down nod of our heads. We were the ones stuck in the tub, huddling there, too afraid to move out of the rising water. This insight fell upon me like a piece of heavy flint on granite stone: it sparked my anger. I had reached my limit of paralysis. The resolve to find a more healing medicine for my husband flared deep within me.

Once kindled, my fight response burned steadily. I marched to the medical college library to research psychoneuroimmunology, attended lectures on Chinese medicine, and read about herbology, meditation, reflexology, homeopathy, and tai chi—I ran through the gamut of alternative health therapies. I even dragged a reluctant Gregg to view a home video of a psychic healing done in the Philippines, a path we decided not to pursue. Sometimes the journey felt foreign, sometimes downright bizarre.

Finally, a friend told us about a doctor who had recently started a practice within a few miles of our home. He was trained in homeopathy, Ayurveda, Chinese and Tibetan medicines, and spiritual counseling. I made an appointment for Gregg. When he returned from his first ninety-minute consultation, I asked how it went.

"It was great," Gregg said.

I plopped into the nearest chair and waited for my backup respiratory system to kick in. Had my husband really uttered these words? For over half a decade, he had approached doctors, needles, and experiments stoically, not wanting to pile his worries upon mine. At long last, a sweet hint of enthusiasm filtered through the gloom. It was as unexpected and out of place as a ray of sunshine during a blizzard. I felt the unmistakable warmth of hope. Could it be, I cautiously questioned, that we were on to something?

Gregg's new treatment consisted primarily of homeopathic remedies, which I knew just as little about as I did Western medicine. Yet we didn't hesitate to try them. After all the needles, experiments, and continued loss of strength, we were very willing to use natural treatments that didn't reek of quackery. During the next six months, Gregg's droopy eyelid, a symptom of myasthenia gravis, improved. The choking ceased. More and more, this path felt right.

About four months into the treatment, his new doctor asked for more information about Gregg's infant and toddler years, so I scrounged up my husband's baby book. Much to my surprise, the doctor said the book increased his understanding of Gregg's disease. Based on those records, he hypothesized that Gregg had had an imbalance in his body from infancy. The allergy shots and medications prescribed through much of his childhood and adolescence may have exacerbated this imbalance, which eventually manifested as a neuropathy. Although no one will ever be able to say for sure why the disease progressed as it did, this was the first explanation of the cause of his illness that we had ever heard. It was comforting.

One day, when I was picking up some remedies for Gregg, his doctor mentioned a seminar he was planning to host in Kathmandu,

Nepal, called *Self-Healing in Ayurvedic and Tibetan Medicines*. I had read a bit about Ayurveda, estimated to be five thousand years old, but had not pursued its practices. Since Nepal was not high on my sightseeing wish list, I didn't give the seminar much thought at first. But then I realized that it would be an opportunity to expand our knowledge, and the more I contemplated the trip, the more compelling the idea became. Soon I fixated on the possibility of going. On one hand, it was totally impractical to consider. I didn't want to schlep a three-year-old and an eight-month-old to a third-world country, but the challenge of finding full-time child care for three weeks felt equally daunting. Also, I doubted whether our employers would approve such an extended absence. On the other hand, I sensed that this adventure might initiate change. It was 1994, and we had been investigating alternative medicine for two years—we needed to keep learning. Much to my surprise, Gregg agreed. I will forever be thankful for the family, friends, and employers who made the trip possible.

The course in Nepal turned out to be the trailhead for our trek into holistic medicine. It was there that we first began to grasp the meaning of "holistic." We did not journey halfway around the world to find a miracle cure, although some family and friends assumed that was our purpose. Instead, we sought a clearer understanding of health and disease, one that would teach us how to take responsibility for our health. During the seminar, we learned why the mind, body, and spirit are inseparable from the disease and healing processes. We gleaned insight into which foods, seasons, climates, and exercises aggravated Gregg's condition, and we compiled a list of remedies used for treating acute illnesses ranging from colds to chicken pox.

We returned home brandishing new confidence and knowledge, which dissolved much of our fear, leaving us free to reconfigure our world. We joined a food co-op and received fresh organic produce every two weeks. We ordered bottled water, retired the microwave to the basement, eliminated chemical cleaners from our home, investigated homeopathy and herbal medicine, and decided, after much thought and research, not to vaccinate our children.

These changes, however, did not happen overnight. Sometimes it took months, sometimes years, to alter a habit or adopt a philosophy. In fact, on the cold January day that I climbed the stairs to the second-floor medicine cabinet, I remembered that it was almost the first anniversary of our trip to Nepal. The changes in our life have been gradual indeed.

Two years into the homeopathic treatments, Gregg decided to check back with his neurologist, whom he had not seen since starting on homeopathic remedies. The neurologist marveled at the neuropathy's slow progression. It would be beyond wonderful if I could report that the neuropathy and all the accompanying disorders have done an about-face. I must admit, however, that Gregg's illness remains a constant challenge. In 1996 we moved to Arizona to escape the cold and damp winters that rendered his hands useless. In 1999 he turned to insulin injections to regulate his blood sugar. Fortunately, Gregg now works full-time, travels frequently for business, golfs (albeit not at his former level), exercises regularly, and coaches our daughters' soccer and softball teams. What we learned—and continue to learn—enables us to support and manage his condition on a daily basis far, far better than we did in the past.

This holistic approach to medicine, which integrates alternative and conventional practices, has blossomed into a holistic approach to life. One of the areas this approach has affected most positively is my parenting experience. At first, I hesitated to use therapies not recommended by our pediatrician. As I researched different Eastern and Western holistic health systems, my fear dissipated; I began to feel comfortable trying the corresponding remedies and treatments. Each time a natural medicine helped heal a fever, sore throat, or ear infection, my trust in the treatment grew. In fact, our youngest daughter has never required an antibiotic even though she has suffered through such illnesses. A holistic approach, however, does not prevent my stomach from turning somersaults when my children are sick. Nor does it preclude using conventional medicine or consulting an M.D. When my daughter severely strained the ligament in her elbow, we made a beeline to the orthopedist.

Our approach to health extends beyond the use of natural remedies. It is a frame of mind, a state of spirit. I am teaching my children how to care for themselves. They are learning the practical. They know, for instance, that ginger tea eases the discomfort of a stomachache and that the homeopathic remedy arnica helps heal a bruise. More important, they are absorbing an attitude toward wellness and disease that I hope they will retain for life. This attitude considers the spiritual, the emotional, the mental, and the physical in all matters of health.

Although the public increasingly seeks alternative medicine in various forms, I have noticed that much of what I use as a parent has not yet been integrated into conventional medicine—especially medicine for children. Not surprisingly, much of the information in this book is rarely discussed in pediatricians' offices. Furthermore, some disciplines, like herbal medicine, are just beginning to be taught in medical schools. In today's world, we parents are pressed for time. We need simple remedies to use when our children become sick. We also need information at our fingertips. My goal is to share the findings of my research, along with my parenting experiences, in order to help fellow parents learn to raise their children in as healthy and holistic an environment as possible.

This book focuses on three user-friendly medicines: herbal medicine, homeopathy, and Ayurveda. The environment, nutrition, vaccinations, and holistic dentistry also receive their due attention. Instead of merely listing recipes for the treatment of illnesses, I strive to impart a deeper understanding of the topic. Where did home-opathy originate? Why doesn't the American Medical Association endorse it? Is it really safe for your children? How, as a parent, do you use it to treat acute illnesses? In addition to the answers to these questions, you will find ideas for transitioning to a healthy, holistic lifestyle.

This book may also serve as a springboard to additional research. The immunization chapter, for instance, may raise your eyebrows or spark some uneasiness; it may not cause you to cease immunizing your child, but it may encourage you to explore the current debate about vaccinations. Likewise, after reading the chapter on organic food, you might not henceforth buy all organic groceries, but you may decide to buy organic produce or dairy products. If questions linger after reading any of the material in the following pages, I en-courage you to investigate the resources listed at the end of the book. Only when you know your options can you make intelligent decisions for yourself and your family.

You do not have to journey to Nepal, as I did, in order to develop a new relationship with health. If you so choose, you can experiment with the principles of holistic health within the comfort of your own home. You need simply to be aware of what's out there. It's like hik-ing through the woods and finding a narrow stream with an out-cropping of rocks just tempting you to try to walk on them. Before you know it, you've rock-hopped to a stable, smooth rock in the middle of the stream. Safe on that rock, you won't topple into the crisp mountain water, yet you can't stand there forever. You have to get to one side or the other. Which side will it be? You've already ex-perienced one side and you're feeling rather curious about the other, so you muster your courage and, with a leap of faith, you land on the opposite shore. As you explore, you discover landscapes and wildflowers that startle you with their beauty. Soon you become adept at jumping between the two sides. You eventually begin to see that the same stream connects them. You have not been exploring two separate worlds, but one interconnected environment.

Do we dare jump across the stones to get to the other side? Whether we have ten, two, or no children, being an adult carries an intrinsic responsibility to show our children how the mind, body, and spirit are connected and how nature plays a stunningly important and beautiful role in each person's life. In our world of cell phones and satellites, of gene manipulation and heart transplants, these concepts can be elusive. In a way, they sound too simple.

The role of every adult, whether a parent or not, is to lead children across life's varied waters. As their guides, especially when the way is not so clear, shouldn't we at least look a little deeper into the world and learn what is beyond our familiar shores, so that we can introduce them to lush, healthful landscapes? Of course we should. But in order to hold out a hand and help them across, we have to venture there first.

CHAPTER 1

So What's Holistic?

The fragmentation of modern life has given rise to a widespread
concern with rediscovering wholeness in human experience.

JOHN WELWOOD, PH.D
REDISCOVERING BASIC WHOLENESS

Earlier in the day, I had arrived at the Ragdale Foundation, an organization in Lake Forest, Illinois, that provides writers, artists, and composers with the space to work independently on projects. I had received a two-week fellowship to start organizing this book. Now, seated for dinner at a long table, the eleven other residents and I engaged in a standard round-robin of introductions. I lived in Arizona, I said, had two children, and was writing a book about holistic parenting. Later, as I was leaving the dining room, another resident, Joan, caught my eye, smiled in a friendly sort of way, and asked, "So what do you mean by 'holistic parenting'?"

I paused at the table where Joan still sat. I had just titled my as-yet-unwritten book *Holistic Parenting* and had not yet been asked this question. About twenty million neurons fired away in my brain, scrounging for an answer. They failed miserably in their mission.

"Well, holistic parenting, ah, you might say, well, you know, takes into consideration the body, mind, and spirit."

Open mouth, insert banality. I shifted my weight to the other foot. Joan's eyebrows remained arched in anticipation of an answer that might generate some interesting dialogue.

Like a pilot of a small aircraft flicking a malfunctioning gauge, I started to panic. My IQ barometric pressure was plummeting. What did holistic mean? How could I describe it? It seemed so complex and yet so simple. I decided to veer around the impending storm before it flung me around like a tumbleweed caught in a desert dust devil.

"Well, for instance, I wrote a sample chapter on vaccinations, not the side you normally hear about, but the adverse side, the one that's starting to attract more attention."

Joan's eyebrows resettled into place. She had young nieces and was interested in this topic.

As I walked back to my room, I rolled the word *holistic* around in my mouth like a cherry Lifesaver. What was its essence—its flavor, scent, and sound? For the next two weeks, in the quiet and solitude of that writers' haven, I pondered this question. I read books on holistic therapy, searched the Web for articles, and jotted down my own thoughts.

Two years later, I'm still savoring the word and probably will do the same tomorrow and every day thereafter. For me, identifying the concepts of *holistic* and integrating them into my life continues to be a step-by-step process. Your experience may be similar. Then again, each of us could experience the meaning of *holistic* in the flash of a moment.

THE WHIMS OF LANGUAGE

Have you noticed how many words simmer in our medical soup pot? The Internet categorizes medicine as conventional, traditional, complementary, integrative, and holistic. Bookstores boast Alternative Health sections. Walk your fingers through the yellow pages and you will discover integrative clinics, holistic clinics, and wellness centers. Do you pick holistic over integrative? Or integrative over alternative? It's almost impossible to make a decision without understanding the terminology.

Language, however, is fickle. Sometimes the word *traditional* refers to a health clinic or hospital; at other times, it refers to the indigenous medicine of a particular culture, such as Native American or Chinese. If you ask your friend what type of medicine the new doctor down the street practices, and she answers "traditional," are you to assume that the doctor primarily uses diagnostic tests and prescription drugs, or that she relies on herbs and acupuncture to help patients heal? Does she assess just your physical health, or is she also concerned about your mental, emotional, and spiritual health?

We muddle meaning. To remedy our confusion, we must create clear definitions. Only then can we ladle out from our soup pot the words that will best help us create a medical model to meet our needs as parents, as human beings, and as guardians of the earth. Understanding what some of our words mean, therefore, is the first step toward understanding what holistic parenting is all about.

Allopathic and Conventional Medicine: One and the Same

I could tell Mary was stressed when she answered the phone.

"What's going on?" I asked.

"I have to take Stephen to the doctor," she said. "He's fussy and feverish. I'm guessing he has an ear infection by the way he's swatting his ear."

My friend bundled up her eighteen-month-old son and went to

see a pediatrician, who inserted an otoscope in little Stephen's ear, noticed an inflammation, and prescribed amoxycillin.

This is an allopathic approach to otitis media, an infection of the middle ear. Allopathy treats disease by "inducing a pathological reaction that is antagonistic to the disease."[1] Antibiotics often are used to create an unfavorable environment for pathogens. These drugs are, in actuality, selective poisons. We hope that the poisoning action is more effective against the bug we want to kill than it is against the patient. Unfortunately, the opposite sometimes happens. Nevertheless, allopathy remains the prevailing approach to illness. It is the medicine that most of us were raised on and still support. It is our convention and our norm.

In certain circumstances allopathy is like the saving kiss upon Snow White's ashen lips. When my four-year-old nephew fell from the top of a high-dive ladder onto the concrete deck, the emergency room physicians and staff saved his life. I would not be around to indulge in an occasional cappuccino but for the blood tests and an appendectomy I received in the seventh grade.

Yet allopathy suffers drawbacks and limitations, too. For one, it is conjoined with the pharmaceutical industry. As such, its chief form of treatment is drugs. Approximately 190 million doses of antibiotics are administered each day in hospitals, while 133 million doses are prescribed each year outside of hospitals.[2] From 1980 to 1992 the use of antibiotics for children jumped 48 percent.[3] Without a doubt, the pharmaceutical industry tremendously influences allopathic medicine.

This relationship breeds some serious side effects. A 1998 study published in the *Journal of the American Medical Association* estimates that adverse drug reactions (ADRs) rank as the sixth leading cause of death, behind heart disease, cancer, stroke, pulmonary disease, and accidents, and just ahead of pneumonia and diabetes.[4] According to this study, approximately 2,216,000 patients hospitalized in 1994 had serious ADRs, and 106,000 had fatal ADRs. These figures don't include patients who experienced ADRs outside hospitals. It is clear from this study that we depend so heavily on synthetic drugs to rid the body of disease that we often overdose on them and consequently poison our bodies, sometimes fatally.

Our readiness to use pharmaceutical drugs, especially antibiotics, not only potentially damages patients, but also damages the medicine itself. The more we use antibiotics, for instance, the less effectively they fight bacteria and viruses. These clever microbes earned their Ph.D. in the art of survival long before the first biochemist donned a mortarboard. Bacteria, we now know, outsmart us by mutating into drug-resistant strains. Our revered ammo—antibiotics—are about as effective as Wile E. Coyote's Acme gunpowder: it doesn't always blow up the right target. From 1992 to 1996 bacterial resistance to ampicillin rose from 29 percent to 38 percent—a 25 percent increase in four short years.[5] When a patient with a life-threatening case of meningitis or pneumonia is whisked into the emergency room, the once effective penicillin may not cure it, nor may multiple classes of backup antibiotics. Such problems have spurred the Centers for Disease Control and Prevention to allocate a whopping $14 million in the year 2000 to its antibiotic-resistance surveillance funds, compared with a paltry $55,000 in 1992.[6]

Perhaps allopathy's greatest weakness is in treating chronic disease. Asthma, arthritis, fibromyalgia, cancer, and AIDS are merely a few of the diseases that stymie researchers. Even chronic childhood ear infections, which have increased 300 percent over the past twenty years, can be added to this list.[7] Weary of the side effects of the medicines used to treat these hard-to-cure diseases, more and more consumers seek other solutions.

Alternative Medicine: The Unconventional

Even before he finished the last dropperful of amoxycillin, Stephen returned to his toddler antics. But one month later—zowee!

"He's got another one," Mary sighed. "It seems like this is a continuation of the last ear infection. Let's see—last time, the doctor prescribed amoxycillin. Now, we have Zithromax. It's supposed to be a stronger antibiotic, so cross your fingers. I need some sleep."

During the next six months, Mary had occasion to repeat these words at least three times, the only variable being the prescription. Finally, with all parties exasperated, the pediatrician referred Stephen to an otolaryngologist, who recommended that tubes be surgically inserted into Stephen's ears. Mary didn't feel relief.

"I'm worried about having him under general anesthesia. I'd feel terrible if something happened," she fretted. "Maybe tubes are the best way to go. The doctor said repeated ear infections can cause hearing loss."

I had recently read about a therapy called cranial sacral manipulation. The article, published in a regional health magazine, mentioned that cranial sacral therapy had treated ear infections effectively and listed some local osteopaths specializing in it. Osteopaths, or D.O.s, receive the same amount of training as medical doctors; both can write prescriptions and perform surgery. The primary difference is that classical osteopaths believe body alignment affects body function. One way to realign the body is to gently move the cranial bones in the skull. Such adjustment may drain the eustachian tube in the middle ear, a theory not yet accepted by conventional medicine. I shared the article with Mary.

"I'm desperate," she said after reading it. "I don't know much about this therapy, but the doctor can see us right away, so I'm going to take the plunge."

Stephen received seven cranial sacral treatments over three weeks. Initially, Mary found the process somewhat time consuming and expensive. However, insurance ended up covering 80 percent of the cost, and the time required for the appointments turned out to be well worth it. After the seventh treatment, the osteopath said Stephen's ears were fine. Mary felt better having a second opinion, so she returned to the otolaryngologist to see if she still recommended tubes for Stephen.

"You're not going to believe this," Mary buzzed over the phone. "I took Stephen to the doctor today and she said his ears are clear. He doesn't need surgery!"

Although no one has determined for sure, I can't help but surmise that the alternative treatment aided the healing process.

The term *alternative medicine* began to percolate in the media in the 1980s and quickly became one of the decade's biggest buzzwords. By 1997 Americans were spending over $27 billion on alternative treatments that included relaxation techniques, herbal medicine, massage, chiropractic, spiritual healing, megavitamins, self-help, guided visualization, lifestyle diet, energy healing, homeopathy, hypnosis, biofeedback, and acupuncture.[8] Most of these modalities, or options, are used to treat chronic illnesses such as arthritis, multiple sclerosis, and asthma, which can plague patients for years on end.

Alternative therapies are here to stay, as evidenced by consumer demand and an increasing insurance coverage of costs incurred from these therapies. Conventional practitioners, however, often remain skeptical of alternative practices. The American Medical Association (AMA) advocates therapies only when their efficiency has been adequately proven by placebo-controlled, double-blind studies. Partially in response to this prerequisite, proponents of alternative therapies, including cranial sacral manipulation, have initiated rigorous testing. A plethora of scientific studies currently focus on herbal medicine. Garlic, ginseng, and echinacea, for instance, receive considerable scrutiny. Other research hinges around modalities like homeopathy and acupuncture. Yet the studies that support some of these medicines don't consume much space on a hard drive. Much more research will be required before organizations like the AMA recommend homeopathy or cranial sacral manipulation to treat common illnesses like middle-ear infections. Nevertheless, the absence of proof doesn't bother the solid base of consumers and medical professionals whose belief in the benefits of alternative medicine is based on personal and clinical experience.

As popular demand pushes alternative therapies closer to the norm, we may need to reconsider the word *alternative,* which implies that a treatment such as homeopathy or acupuncture is second string, serving as backup and coming into play only when the first-string treatment—conventional medicine—cannot perform. Why not include all of our options in the first-string treatment? The opponents of alternative medicine may bristle at this suggestion, but it sounds like fair play to me.

COMPLEMENTARY AND INTEGRATIVE MEDICINE: ALMOST ONE AND THE SAME

Complementary Medicine

Had Stephen seen a physician practicing complementary medicine, a referral to a specialist like an osteopath would not have been unusual. The word *complementary* implies that at least two systems—in this case, conventional and alternative medicine—coexist side by side.

The use of the word *complementary* to describe medicine began in

Britain, where such practice is now respected and commonplace. In the United States, the word crops up within the acronym CAM, which stands for Complementary and Alternative Medicine. In February 1999 the National Institutes of Health transformed the seven-year-old Office of Alternative Medicine into the National Center for Complementary and Alternative Medicine (NCCAM). The NCCAM researches alternative therapies and disseminates information to the public and to health care professionals. Projects funded with the NCCAM's $50 million-plus budget include studies of the effects of massage on premature infants, the ability of garlic to lower cholesterol, the ability of echinacea to prevent and treat upper respiratory infections and chronic ear problems in children, and the efficacy of bee-sting therapy to treat multiple sclerosis.

Integrative Medicine: A Synthesis

Integrative and complementary medicines are very similar. "Integrative," however, has a more inclusive ring to it, meaning that the various types of medicine, from allopathic to alternative, are meshed together. Rather than sitting side by side, the disciplines become parts of a singular system. Practitioners of integrated medicine have a gamut of therapies at their fingertips.

One of the best examples of the practice of integrative medicine is the Program in Integrative Medicine at the University of Arizona College of Medicine, Tucson. Dr. Andrew Weil, the best-selling author of *Spontaneous Healing* and *Eating Well for Optimum Health,* established this program in 1996. I spoke with one of the fellows in Weil's program, who began her practice in a large health maintenance organization (HMO). There, her appointments with patients averaged only fifteen minutes; now, her patient consultations average an hour. For a child with chronic middle-ear infections, she may recommend homeopathic remedies, herbs, or dietary changes such as the elimination of dairy products. Surgically inserted ear tubes may be a last resort of treatment although it depends on the individual case. For acute ear infections involving extreme pain or high fever, she may turn to an antibiotic.

Besides promoting integrative medicine, Weil focuses on the role of physicians as teachers. Whether allopathic or alternative, doctors must teach patients appropriate self-care techniques. When ill, patients can then initiate their medical care rather than passively rely on a professional. If a child comes down with an ear infection, for example, a parent will know what steps to take at home to begin the healing process. The burden placed on ambulatory clinics and hospital emergency rooms, especially during cold and flu seasons, will ease, and insurance companies will pay fewer claims.

The first time I visited an integrative physician, I was thrown for a loop. I arrived at the appointment eager to discuss the possibility of being weaned from thyroid medication. Although the doctor inquired about my physical health, he also asked what I did for a living, how I liked my career, what time I went to bed, how much coffee and soda I drank, what role religion played in my life, and what my relationships with family members were like. In the past, I had never spent more than twenty or thirty minutes at a doctor's appointment, nor had I encountered a physician whose questions about my health extended beyond the physical. This time, the doctor addressed the intangible—my emotions, feelings, habits, and beliefs—as well as the tangible. I must admit that revealing such intimate information felt strange. Yet talking to a compassionate listener about the details of my life was a satisfying experience. A special relationship began to develop during that first ninety-minute appointment.

HOLISTIC MEDICINE, HOLISTIC LIFE

So how is holistic medicine different from integrative medicine? For the most part, actually, the words *holistic* and *integrative* are interchangeable. Both connote medicine that appraises the patient's physical, emotional, mental, and spiritual health and then treats the whole person.

I prefer the word *holistic,* however, because it reminds me of the internal and the external, the visible and the invisible, the near and the far. I may live in the desert, but the desert overlaps the mountains, which slope into the ocean, which connects me to other lands, which harbor humans who contain atoms, molecules, cells, organs, feelings, ego, soul, and spirit. The tapestry of life is intricate and vast. As each of us weaves the unique details of an individual life into this tapestry, our lives become connected. The person who experiences the world holistically is acutely aware that everyone weaves together using the same raw materials. This rare individual feels, tastes, smells, hears, and sees the interrelatedness and interdependence of all things, great and small.

Our health is also woven into this tapestry. Every thread from our society, culture, environment, food, relationships, and emotions influences us to some degree. Medicine, therefore, must take into account all these factors as it strives to help us restore or maintain our balance. As Harriet Beinfield and Efrem Korngold say in their book *Between Heaven and Earth: A Guide to Chinese Medicine,* "Medicine not only defines health and disease, but also makes implicit assumptions about what life is and what it is to be human."[9] In order for medicine to make these assumptions, it must consider the whole of life. Holistic medicine reflects a holistic approach to life.

This book explores concepts of holistic living. You will find many easy-to-use ideas that foster a natural and simple lifestyle. Implement the ideas that appeal to you. Bear in mind that you do not need to make changes within a certain time frame or in a certain order. Rather, what you need to do is savor the changes you make as you would savor a cherry Lifesaver, and decide if their flavor satisfies you. This is how to learn what holistic living is all about. You then can decide whether you are comfortable with its concepts and practices, and whether you want your child to know and experience them, too.

My experiences have led me to believe that a holistic lifestyle is the healthiest legacy that I can pass on to my children. As a parent, you decide what is best for your child.

CHAPTER 2

The Fear of It All

Fear is the destructive energy in man. It withers the mind, it
distorts thought, it leads to all kinds of extraordinarily clever and
subtle theories, absurd superstitions, dogmas, and beliefs.

KRISHNAMURTI

With a medicine cabinet devoid of synthetic remedies, a kitchen cabinet overflowing with herbs and spices, and a refrigerator stocked with organic food, I felt that our family had embraced a holistic lifestyle fairly well. Then I contracted a virus. I suffered through an entire week of fever and lethargy during which I headquartered on the couch by day and ordered pizza by night. Yes, I know—real holistic.

After a few fever-free days, my joints started swelling. First my wrists, then my fingers, then my knees and toes. My concern ballooned right along with my joints until it inflated into a big ball of worry. The symptoms were the same as those my cousin had when he was diagnosed with Lyme disease. Having recently reveled in northern Minnesota's wooded wonderland, a haven for deer ticks, I wanted to be tested for Lyme. My homeopath, however, prescribed the wait-and-see approach. Not being in the wait-and-see mood, I went to visit an allopathic family physician, who thought my symptoms might be a secondary reaction to the virus; he prescribed a dose of wait-and-see, too, but authorized a Lyme test anyway. Perhaps this second reassuring pat on the hand calmed me because I decided to let nature run its course. I never did complete the blood test.

When my joints and I settled down, I realized that my actions had been motivated by fear. I slid from a space of certainty to one of the unknown, which, in essence, is the pit of fear. I was scared. This happens to all of us, of course, but I was somewhat taken aback by this fear. During the previous five years, I had discovered that knowledge eases fear; the more I learned about health issues and the more I experimented with sound remedies, the less frightened I was by disease. Yet here I was again, face-to-face with my old acquaintance: fear.

THE FACES OF FEAR

I once heard a pastor say that there are two constants in this world, fear and love, and that every emotion, reaction, and relationship stems from them. If this theory is true, then fear will continue to tap-dance alongside us. This doesn't mean that we must be fear's Ginger Rogers or Fred Astaire. We can always choose a different dance partner. But that's difficult to do when we are caught up in the beat hovering over the parquet floor.

As parents, we often brush against fear. I was hanging out with a group of moms and kids once when one of the women confessed the incredible love she had for her child and how she worried about the many traumas he could suffer. "I don't even let myself think about those things," another mother piped up. When her mind wandered into the danger zone, she redirected it. As a psychotherapist friend told me, one of the finest gifts of love to a child is a parent who can find her own serenity.

One way to cultivate such serenity is to look our fears in the face and determine whether they are justified or irrational. One of our baby-sitters had a great fear of bees. This fear stuck like honey to our preschooler. When an errant yellow jacket flew into our car, our daughter clapped her hands in a panic and sandwiched the unfortunate victim between her palms. She got stung, of course, which only exacerbated her fear. Children tend to absorb the fears of the adults around them, be those fears reasonable or unreasonable.

To be sure, some fears are justified. These are natural, almost instinctual fears, like the fear of physical danger. This fear prompts me to keep my kids out of the desert during snake season. Determining what is and isn't safe, however, can be a hard call to make. We don't want to encourage serious injury, nor do we want to inhibit moderate risk taking.

Our own experience figures significantly in our judgment concerning our children's safety, as it did when my seven-year-old fetched me so that I could watch her ride her bike over a 2-foot jump.

"But I just did it, Mama!" she said when I expressed concern.

"Well, she's wearing her helmet," I thought. "Let's see what happens." I remembered surviving a few bike tumbles in childhood. With bated breath, I watched her pedal down the hill, up the ramp, and complete a wipeout that ranked a solid 9.5. She still has a scar on her side from the abrasion. Needless to say, she hasn't attempted any more jumps, and I haven't encouraged her to do so, although, if she wanted to, I would reluctantly give my consent.

Another instinctive fear assails me when my children get sick. As the thermometer's mercury rises, a certain uneasiness swells in my solar plexus and spreads with every breath. I'm now resigned to this phenomenon, but I recognize it for what it is: a reflex that heightens my senses. Like every parent, I don't enjoy when my nervous system zooms to the Defcon 4 level of alertness. Yet, being alert helps me slow down and carefully observe the young patient, who then receives the extra attention so needed during illness.

It used to be that when my children became sick, I felt compelled to give them medicine as soon as possible. Like my daughter with bees, I felt panicky. God forbid that the fever shoot out of control or strep throat turn into rheumatic fever. Rather than allowing nature the slightest opportunity to do her thing, my knee-jerk reaction was to reach for the orange-flavored acetaminophen, which was the only remedy I knew. It gave both me and my children the "temporary relief" promised on the label.

Ironically, my children are not frightened when they're sick. Remember being sick as a child? Those nasty colds and flus were miserable, but I never was afraid that I would die or have a febrile seizure because of a high fever. I just felt lousy. Even when the doctor determined that my appendix had to come out, I wasn't frightened. I was relieved that the pain would end. When ill, I wanted to feel better. I also wanted my mom, the soft quilt with the tiny violets on it, and my own bed. In fact, even now when I'm all stuffed up and run down, my mother's voice still makes me feel better.

Fear protects, yet fear distorts. It is not something to grind up in the garbage disposal or shoo into the pantry. We need fear as much as we need the nerve endings in our hands to tell us when the pots in the dishwasher are still too hot to remove. Problems arise, however, when we allow our fears to gallop away unbridled. That's when we create adversity.

The Problems We Create

In a world hit hard by cancer, AIDS, diabetes, and hundreds of other now incurable diseases, fear is hard to quell. Most of the time, we don't even attempt to do so. Whether we're aware of it or not, we excel at feeding our fears, not starving them. Newspapers, radio talk shows, TV news, and magazines all feed our anxieties. Titles like "Flesh-Eating Strep and Food Tainting *E. Coli* Aren't the Only Strains to Fear" and "Fever Facts: When to Worry, What to Do" keep us skittish. Movies thrill us with plots about deadly viruses escaping test tubes and threatening mankind's existence. No wonder that when our children get sick, our imaginations take off like a missile, with a trajectory that leads to nightmares of disability or death.

This malaise of fear generates some serious side effects, one of which brings us back to the antibiotic problem. One reason that doctors overprescribe antibiotics is because patients or, in the case of children, the parents demand the medicine. In a study of six hundred pediatricians, 96 percent of doctors reported that parents requested antibiotics for children who had viral colds or upper respiratory infections. Nearly one-quarter of parents asked for a specific drug. Moreover, one-third of doctors admitted that they complied with these parents' demands even when they knew that the drug would be ineffective.[1]

I can understand why parents demand antibiotics. I've done it myself. At four months old, my daughter developed thrush, a fungal infection of the mouth that causes mild discomfort. The pediatrician prescribed an antibiotic, which I religiously administered to the very last drop. The thrush remained obstinate. The doctor ordered another prescription, but the characteristic white spots persisted. Since the spots made me nervous, I was fully prepared to renew the prescription. I didn't know what else to do; I knew of no other options for treatment. When the pediatrician hesitated to honor my request, we discussed in detail the option of going without treatment. The doctor helped me feel confident that my baby's mouth would heal over time, which is exactly what it did.

In a study published in the *Journal of the American Medical Association,* physicians estimated that antibiotic prescriptions for upper respiratory tract infections, which account for three-quarters of drug prescriptions written in doctors' offices, could safely be reduced by 10 to 30 percent.[2] The study concluded that doctors too often yield to parents' demands for antibiotics, and that parents would be less inclined to insist on antibiotics if a physician, nurse, or other medical professional educated them about their child's illness and the healing process. Parents want reassurance that their child's bad cold will not progress into a more serious illness such as pneumonia.

The Centers for Disease Control and Prevention has combined efforts with state health agencies, HMOs, and professional organizations like the American Association of Pediatrics and the American Academy of Family Physicians to create educational materials for physicians and parents. The purpose of these materials is to decrease the number of needless prescriptions and, accordingly, the bacterial resistance to antibiotics.

"Yuck! You've Got Germs"

The fear of virulent strains of pathogens lurking around has made us germ-phobic. We are obsessed with obliterating germs because we fear the diseases that we think they cause. Over seven hundred antibacterial products have inundated the market since 1992.[3] Antibacterial soap now appears as a staple on my children's school supply list, but a squirt a day doesn't keep all bacteria away. Remember, these pathogens are smart. They can mutate into more virulent strains that exacerbate our problems. A little old-fashioned soap and water would be more than sufficient for the kids to use before lunch. My dish towel even came bearing a sticker that said "Anti-Microbial," which I assume is supposed to make me feel safer in the kitchen. The towel's finish protects against the growth of bacteria.

My daughter Hannah gave a partially eaten Popsicle to my daughter Elle, who turned up her nose at it. "Elle, you don't want to eat it because you're afraid you'll get my yucky germs," Hannah declared. Through osmosis, through just hanging out in society, Hannah had absorbed this notion.

A Few Solutions

We fear germs. As a result, we wage indiscriminate war against a microscopic population that is older than dinosaur bones. We fear disease. When we fall sick, our knee-jerk reaction often is to eliminate the symptoms as quickly as possible. How do we tame this fear-fed frenzy? Fear will never disappear, but perhaps we can reduce it to a reasonable level.

Fair warning: this task is challenging. It primarily involves the mind, which has been known to play all sorts of havoc with reality. This trickster creates thoughts that have the ability to trip from one person to another like dominos falling in a line. If enough of the same thoughts settle into everyone's minds, society develops a collective consciousness that can be difficult to alter. Right now, our collective consciousness quivers at the mention of germs or disease.

As I see it, three things can help us mitigate our fears: awareness, knowledge, and experience.

Awareness

First, take time to observe the fear plastered on billboards, written into magazine articles, and headlined on television. Learn to identify worst-case scenarios. These are the tales of horror and woe that besiege us in doctor's offices, day cares, schools, and during chats with neighbors. These stories skew reality.

Chicken pox recently has become a focus of worst-case-scenario fears. Before the advent of the chicken pox vaccine, three to four million cases of varicella zoster virus (chicken pox) occurred in the

United States each year. Approximately ten thousand cases required hospitalization, and about one hundred cases resulted in death. In the adults and children who died, secondary infections, particularly strep, had often set in and proved to be fatal.

Millions of children, however, have survived chicken pox, which was once perceived as an innocuous rite of childhood but is now regarded as a serious and potentially fatal illness that should be expunged. One mother said to me, "My doctor said I shouldn't risk letting my kids get chicken pox." Chicken pox hasn't changed; just our perception of it has. Yet some medical philosophies, like Traditional Chinese Medicine, believe that chicken pox strengthens the immune system and therefore is a productive disease, not one to eliminate.

We must also be aware of how we use words. We are more inclined to *fight* disease, *combat* cancer, and *destroy* bacteria than we are to *learn* from disease, *work* with illness, *support* the body, and *heal*. Pay attention to language. Children inhale the words we exhale.

Have you ever overheard a nervous parent say something like this? *"Do you think I should take Sarah to a doctor? She's really congested, and I was up with her four times last night. She's kind of feverish. I'm worried that she has an ear infection."*

I've said these words. Who knows what message my daughter picked up from them? Does she think that sickness is something to worry about? That someone besides her mom or dad must help her get better? That her ear infection is a scary, serious condition? Yes, sickness can be frightening and scary, but we need to give our bodies the opportunity to do what they were designed to do, which is heal themselves. As one holistic doctor told me, the body always responds in the most appropriate way possible at any given moment. Fevers, for instance, create an environment hostile to bacteria and viruses and are thus a healing mechanism. The body may need the support of medicine during the healing process; however, "support" does not mean "suppress." Herbal medicines and homeopathy help reduce fevers without suppressing them. Many herbal remedies can easily be made at home. We simply need to know what the remedies are. We need knowledge.

Knowledge

Knowledge displaces ignorance. It empowers us to take action. If we know how to safely and effectively begin treating ear infections, then before taking Sarah or Sam to the doctor, we will turn to nonprescription therapies like olive-oil-and-garlic ear drops or homeopathic remedies. Knowledge gives us options; options enable us to assume responsibility for our health.

In today's information age, acquiring knowledge is easier than opening a can of soup, provided we have the time and inclination to gather it. Health food stores and co-ops usually are well stocked with local and national publications brimming with information on alternative medicine. Monthly newsletters such as *Mothers & Others for a Liveable Planet* print interesting, solidly researched articles, as well as provide a host of resources and references. In addition, tons of Internet information is just a few clicks away.

Ironically, once we have knowledge, we may experience new fears and frustrations. Suddenly, we know that we don't know, so we search and learn; as we learn, we move into new territory, a very disconcerting feeling indeed. We are as disoriented as a small child desperately searching for his parents among a sea of legs at Disney World. Feeling disoriented alarms us and often sends us fleeing to known ground. We need to stay put, however, in order to work through our fear or frustration. Otherwise, we never learn or grow.

One of the most frustrating learning processes I have experienced involved vaccinations. When I researched the vaccine chapter for this book, I was overwhelmed with information. Although I eventually chose to present one side of the issue, I gathered information about both the pros and cons of immunizations. Sorting through the persuasive arguments on each side was a gargantuan task. It left me terribly frustrated. All I could do was read, sort, and digest the information. Eventually, I concluded that vaccinations did not fit into my paradigm of health. Part of my decision not to vaccinate my children was based on scientific studies and clinical experiences that point to the dangers and deficiencies of vaccines. Rather than subject my children to substances that present clear risks—which we will discuss later—I chose to rely on a holistic standard of health. I based another part of my decision on intuition. As I created a more holistic lifestyle, the idea of vaccinating my children no longer felt right.

Intuition is a source of knowledge we are not taught to heed. In her book *Awakening Intuition: Using Your Mind-Body Network for Insight and Healing,* Dr. Mona Lisa Shulz writes, "For most of us, the first step toward hearing the language of intuition requires that we become open to accepting another, seemingly illogical way of perceiving and receiving information."[5] She describes the strong role intuition plays in her private medical practice and how she has observed its use within the medical field, particularly by nurses.

Intuition is a great asset, but so often in parenting we ignore its wisdom. As my friend David Russell writes in his book *The Names of Life,* "We often turn away, shy of the mystic within us, or dispute our own wisdom, content with the lesser path of secondhand knowledge."[6] We may surrender to the knowledge of "experts" even if their opinions conflict with our inner knowing.

When five-year-old Michael fell and hurt his arm on the playground, the school nurse saw that he could move his arm, so she reassured him that he was okay and sent him back to class. Later that day, a tearful Michael, complaining of pain, returned to the nurse's office. When his mother arrived at the school, the nurse reiterated that nothing was broken. By 8:00 P.M., Michael's mother felt that something was wrong, despite the fact that Michael could move his arm. Her intuition told her to take her son to the emergency room. X rays confirmed a break.

We must continuously pay attention to our intuition and allow it to guide us. It should not replace book knowledge; rather, it should be used in conjunction with it. Unfortunately, there are no definite rules about when to trust intuition. We have to practice listening to and following our inner wisdom, which, more often than not, tells us what is best for our child.

Experience

Like knowledge, experience dilutes fear. "In all cases, there is a reciprocity between experience and knowledge—knowledge interprets our experiences while experience enriches our knowledge," says Dr. Eric Cassell in his book *The Nature of Suffering*.[7] If a therapy or medicine isn't proven by a double-blind study and published in a reputable medical journal, we often remain leery of it, even if clinical experience has repeatedly demonstrated the therapy's or medicine's effectiveness. We want definitive explanations that can be written in textbooks and taught to professionals, who then become responsible for making us well. We want guarantees.

You can read all you want about homeopathy or herbal medicines, but you will never know how they really work until you try them. If you're looking for a step-by-step way to get into holistic medicine or to create a holistic lifestyle, you probably won't find one. I can't tell you exactly how to do it. Some people, like me, try it out of desperation. Others experience a feeling of discontent, a feeling that other options exist outside the realm of conventional medicine. They want to assume the responsibility of healing, not turn it over to someone else. Curiosity, or maybe a sense of adventure, drives others to experience alternative therapies. Perhaps in your exploration, you will try an herbal or homeopathic remedy first, or maybe you will begin with an organic diet low in sugar, salt, and additives. I can point you in the right direction and suggest how to make such changes, but ultimately you are the one who will have to try the new medicine or new lifestyle. No one can experience it for you.

CHAPTER 3

Health and Medicine
Across the Ages

In holism, ancient and modern systems and technologies can
complement one another in a cohesive and universal manner.

DENNIS K. CHERNIN, M.D.
HOLISTIC MEDICINE: ITS GOALS, MODELS, AND HISTORICAL ROOTS

In the spring of 1999, Dr. Andrew Weil and Dr. Arnold Relman, editor-in-chief emeritus of the *New England Journal of Medicine*, debated on national television the validity of integrative medicine. Dr. Relman expressed a concern that integrating alternative therapies into medicine would cause confusion in medical school curriculums and would contradict the foundation on which modern medicine rests. He also said that alternative methods have not been adequately proven by the gold standard of controlled, randomized clinical trials. Furthermore, while acknowledging the role of the mind in psychosomatic diseases, Relman questioned the mind's ability to heal disease.

Dr. Weil, on the other hand, reiterated the belief that he has expressed in many of his books: that the mind can abet the body's innate healing processes. Not all therapies, Weil said, must be justified by double-blind studies. Clinical experience also should be allowed to validate them. Weil pointed out that the Office of Technology Assessment of the U.S. Congress estimates that less than 30 percent of procedures used by conventional medicine have been rigorously tested. In addition, he said, data supporting many alternative therapies is "scattered in far-flung places" and must be compiled for - evaluation. Just because this information has not been gathered or studied does not mean it is erroneous.

Whether you side with Relman or Weil, if you had heard the entire debate, you certainly would agree that these two doctors represent opposing views that are prevalent within today's medical arena. Neither one of these belief systems, or paradigms, spontaneously developed from thin air; like all paradigms, they evolved over time. Despite their differences, the paradigms have at least one thing in common: the same historical background. If you think about it, we all share the same history. Hippocrates, Chinese medicine, Pasteur, the germ theory, and Jonas Salk are part of everyone's historical background, regardless of what you believe about health. The only variable to this shared history is in the interpretation of its meaning.

If we all share a common history, and if all present beliefs evolve from this history, then examining history will give us a better understanding of our current medicines. If the history in this next section gives you a case of the yawns, I suggest skipping it. In other words, don't get bogged down here; move on to more current events. I chose to include this section because comparing foreign systems of medicine within a historical context has afforded me insight into the effectiveness and safety of those medicines, some of which I use. A certain confidence and security comes from knowing that the science of Chinese medicine and the science of Ayurveda have been employed skillfully for thousands of years and are still practiced today in many parts of the world, including the United States and Europe.

A VERY CONDENSED VIEW OF HISTORY

Our journey from past to present is going to resemble a stone skipping across the time line of history. We'll touch down in five places, which will be enough to understand how our conventional and alternative medicines evolved. As we point our binoculars toward the past, we must remember that our feet remain solidly planted in our culture. From this modern-day perspective, the ideas, beliefs, and customs of bygone times can feel mighty strange and uncomfortable. The ancient Chinese, Egyptians, and Greeks didn't have a Nintendo to their names, but they were sophisticated in many other ways. When we integrate the wisdom and the achievements of past eras into our current culture and everyday life, our health and medical systems will benefit.

Traditional Chinese Medicine: 2500 B.C. to Present

The first introduction I had to Traditional Chinese Medicine (TCM) was a lecture. Nothing unusual happened until about halfway through when the instructor asked me to stick out my tongue. After examining the color, coating, and cracks, he proceeded to tell me about various imbalances in my body. Practitioners of TCM often use tongue diagnosis to determine the health of internal organs.

Traditional Chinese Medicine has been in use for over two thousand years, yet at first glance it looks about as plausible as Rumpelstiltskin spinning straw into gold. The concept of *chi* (pronounced "CHEE" and sometimes spelled *qi*) seems particularly strange. Chi is often described as the life force or the vital energy present in all living systems. This energy moves throughout the body on pathways, or channels, called meridians that extend through every tissue and organ of the body, almost like a secondary nervous system. Disturbances in the proper movement of chi may prevent the body from functioning properly.

Chi is like the electricity in a lightbulb. You can't see electricity, but you know it is present when light emanates from the bulb. When electricity is blocked or shut off, it no longer travels along the bulb's filament and generates light. Chi, the bioelectrical energy of the body, travels through us in a similar way. Our bodies' tissues and organs are like the filament and other physical components of the bulb. When chi is blocked, inhibited, or shut off, it cannot enter our tissues and organs. Our bodies then either malfunction or die.

Practitioners locate disturbed chi using a variety of diagnostic techniques, such as tongue, iris, skin, and nail diagnosis, and even pulse diagnosis, in which twenty-eight different pulse positions on a person's wrists are used to determine the health of organs and bodily functions. Treatments for disturbed chi include acupuncture, a technique in which needles are inserted into particular meridian points to stimulate the movement of chi; herbal medicines, which also enter meridian pathways and affect chi; special forms of massage; and exercises such as tai chi or chi kong.

Traditional Chinese Medicine attributes the cause of illness to blocked chi, not to the presence of viruses, bacteria, or other pathogens. When chi is blocked along the kidney or gallbladder meridians, for example, which both run through the ear, immunity decreases. The middle ear, or other points along the meridian, may become infected with viruses or other microbes. Furthermore, climatic factors affect chi. Cold wind and cold weather can influence the chi in the ear and lead to middle-ear infections. Factors like suppressed emotions, rich or spicy foods, and overeating can unbalance the flow of chi in the liver and gallbladder, as can an excess of sugar, dairy, and gluten, all of which are phlegm-producing foods. Otitis media, an infection of the middle ear, can result from such an imbalance. As mentioned, acupuncture stimulates the flow of chi and is therefore effective in treating ear infections as well as infectious diseases like sinusitis and pneumonia, which also result from chi blockages.[1]

In TCM, the whole must be understood before the parts can be understood. A disorder of the ear, for example, such as otitis media, cannot be treated without considering the spleen or the kidney because these organs are functionally connected to the ear. TCM does not require specialists who concentrate on only one system or organ of the body; the same physician treats a person for all illnesses. The body is seen as an entity whose individual parts work together in particular patterns. Treating one part and ignoring other parts could easily lead to misdiagnosis or mistreatment.

Within the whole there are parts, but each part embodies the whole. Think of it this way: Each human is a microcosm of the macrocosmic universe. If both you and I are miniature universes, then we share the same energies—or the same chi—with the atmosphere, the ozone layer, the rain forests, and lakes, rivers, plants, and animals. When the energy of any of these changes, our energy also changes, be it for better or worse. As you are probably noticing, this concept is very foreign to our Western consciousness.

Sometimes I wonder what my life would be like if I had grown up with TCM. How would I regard my body? How would I handle acute illness? How would my reactions to everyday stresses differ?

What would I see in my children?

Hippocrates: 460–377 B.C.

Moving west and up the time line, we encounter Hippocrates, who is regarded as the father of Western medicine and is referred to in many books as the father of holistic medicine, as well. Many a physician still quotes his golden rule: "First, do no harm." Graduating medical students take the Hippocratic oath, which is based on his philosophies. Ironically, some of Hippocrates' holistic beliefs and practices have fallen from the auspices of modern medicine.

Hippocrates recognized, as did the entire Greek culture, that a certain harmony exists within all systems of the universe. Disregarding the rhythms of this harmony, he reasoned, unbalances a person's physical, emotional, mental, and spiritual health. Dr. Henry Skolimowksi comments on this concept in his essay "Wholeness, Hippocrates, and Ancient Philosophy":

> By extending this insight ever so slightly, we might say that illness is the result of holding a wrong philosophy, one which permits one to behave foolishly and disharmoniously, one which does not help one to perceive the body and the mind as a whole.[2]

Hippocrates, for example, advocated that humans live in accordance with the seasons. He believed that "with the seasons, the digestive organs of men undergo a change."[3] Eating foods harmonious with the season, as well as the climate, helps balance one's health. We recognize this philosophy when we gravitate to beef stew or chili during the winter. In January, watermelon may tempt us in the supermarket, but Hippocrates would advocate avoiding the temptation. Consuming summer fruits during cold months contradicts nature's rhythm and interferes with proper digestion.

Hippocrates also believed that one's environment influences the healing process. The Grecian center of healing, called an aesclepion, resembled our modern-day health spas more than it did our hospitals. Natural settings, filled with plants and birds and moist, earthy smells, encouraged lengthy recuperative stays and helped restore balance to the body, mind, and spirit. Each aesclepion boasted beautiful temples where patients went for healing ceremonies. In fact, the Greeks gave the spiritual side of healing more attention than the physical side.

Of the three hundred aesclepia, the most famous was on the island of Kos, Hippocrates' birthplace. Here, some six thousand herbs were available to practitioners. Although the Grecian pharmacy was well equipped, Hippocrates felt that medicine would be weak if only drugs were used to achieve cures. He preached that nature cures most illness.

Hildegard of Bingen: A.D. 1098–1179

Parallels to TCM and Hippocratic medicine emerge, surprisingly, in the Middle Ages in the work of Saint Hildegard of Bingen. Hildegard was a Benedictine nun, abbess, mystic, musician, preacher, prophet, poet, natural historian, theologian, and scientist. Her extensive written legacy includes books, symphonias, and illustrations, as well as vast correspondence with political and religious leaders of the time. Today, you can purchase CDs of her chants and symphonias at major bookstores and music stores.

Even though she lacked professional medical training, Hildegard's medicine deserves our attention. As a mystic, she received information through visions. Her medicine reflects her faith in God and her recognition that the Divine illuminates the human spirit. Like Hippocrates, Saint Hildegard teaches that through our connection with Spirit we can access our innate healing powers. Our inner wisdom is often as precise as studies and experiences in the material world. Everything on Earth is available to help us on our journey of life, in times of good health and ill health. We just need to learn how to use plants, fruits, minerals, and animals as we make this journey. Hildegard's writings explain how to do this.

Her book *Physica* is a handbook of remedies, while *Causae et Curae* ("Causes and Cures") is a detailed medical text. These books describe in detail how emotions and lifestyle influence one's health. A dysfunctional liver, for instance, creates an imbalance called "black bile," which in turn unbalances the emotions, making one melancholic or angry. To prevent black bile, Hildegard espoused a proper diet that promotes proper digestion, thereby supporting the liver. Like Hippocrates, she believed that food is medicinal. Spelt, for example, a type of wheat grain that is used in over two thousand Hildegard recipes, is an easily digested alkaline grain that counteracts the high amounts of acids found in many of today's foods. It is appearing more frequently in health food stores and restaurants.

In 1993 Dr. Wighard Strehlow started the Hildegard Practice, a clinic located near Lake Constance in western Germany. Here, doctors use Hildegard's herbs, recipes, and lifestyle recommendations to treat patients with heart disorders, cancer, rheumatoid arthritis, depression, and a host of other illnesses. Dr. Strehlow explains:

> Out of God's wisdom, Hildegard medicine has perhaps been reserved for the helplessness of our times. It is so modern that only now, with our scientific knowledge of medicine, can we begin to appreciate Hildegard's remarkable understanding of the basic causes of health and sickness.[4]

René Descartes: 1596–1650

In the 1600s, the West focused on a new approach to the world. A French philosopher, mathematician, and physicist named René Descartes, famed for his statement "I think, therefore I am," catalyzed this shift in perspective with the development of a new scientific philosophy. Descartes wanted to construct a science that explained nature with absolute proof and certainty. In his *Discourse on the Method of Rightly Conducting the Reason, and Seeking Truth in the Sciences,* Descartes writes, "We reject all knowledge which is merely probable and judge that only those things should be believed which are perfectly known and about which there can be no doubts."[5] This doctrine, now called the Cartesian philosophy, continues to strongly influence our thinking and behavior.

Although agreeing with Hildegard that God exists, Descartes preached that rational thought leads to the truth. Rationalism, which depends on intellect and logical reasoning, replaced spirituality as the favored method for ascertaining reality. Descartes viewed humans as the supreme beings of reason. As such, they controlled all that they observed, including nature. Consequently, nature was an entity separate from people, who possessed the reason and intellect to overpower it. Today, we still attempt to conquer nature.

Descartes also bequeathed us analytical reasoning. This led to the philosophy that in order to understand the whole, science should first dissect and analyze the parts. All of nature, including the human body, was now portrayed as a finely tuned machine. Probing each part of the machine led to an understanding of the whole. The body could not possibly be fathomed without first understanding its individual components. This thinking, of course, is the antithesis of TCM and Hippocratic medicine, which never dissect the whole into parts but study systems and patterns instead.

Conventional medicine still uses the language of machinery to describe the body. Now fragmented into a plethora of specialties, this medicine is a Cartesian legacy. If our hearts go haywire, the mechanic of this organ, a cardiologist, tries to repair them. Our continued fascination with the pieces of the body has resulted in the Human Genome Project. Initiated in 1990 by the National Institutes of Health, the Department of Energy, and various European labs, it has sequenced 300 million base pairs of DNA in order to locate approximately 100,000 human genes. By pinpointing the genes involved in particular diseases, like Parkinson's disease or breast cancer, scientists hope to determine who is at risk for the disease, detect it at an early stage, and develop very precise drugs to defeat it. Although this sounds magnificent in its technical sophistication, we can't disregard the effects that a person's spiritual strength, way of dealing with emotions, and manner of caring for the physical body have on the disease process.

Twentieth-Century Quantum Physics

Although the Cartesian model tremendously influences our perception of health and disease, some quantum physicists have deviated to a different view of life. Albert Einstein catalyzed this shift with his theory of relativity, which states that matter and energy are one, and that they are constantly in a state of flux. Energy becomes matter and matter becomes energy. At no point are they static.

This theory may be a little confusing to understand when you first hear it. After all, most of us grew up learning that the universe is made up of particles that can be isolated, weighed, and measured. Now, some scientists contend that the universe is not made up of particles, nor is it made up of energies that don't have any specific form. Rather, the universe is a continual event of inter-evolving transmutations between energy and matter. Whew, that's a mouthful, isn't it?

To make this idea a little less complicated, think of the universe as a dynamic place that constantly changes. (Just be aware that this greatly oversimplifies the quantum issue, which is still being debated within physics.) This dynamic world is full of creative, spontaneous energy events, which impact our health positively or negatively. If mainstream medicine someday acknowledges the role that such energy events play in health and disease, it will have to stop looking solely at what can be weighed and measured with machines. So far, our machines can't weigh and measure energy events.

The implications of such quantum theories are nothing less than astounding and radical. Although biochemistry, genetics, and conventional medicine will continue to be studied and used, energy will one day play a more prominent role in medical science. Energy will be recognized as having the ability to heal the body. This recognition will validate alternative therapies like therapeutic touch and acupuncture, as well as various types of body work, including Reiki and Shiatsu, which utilize the body's innate energy systems. Moreover, the mind will be considered capable of moving energy and therefore matter. Therapies like visualization and meditation will be better understood. As we begin to accept and work with the forces of the universe, our spiritual awareness will be heightened.

For now, the concept of energy remains outside the boundaries of conventional medicine. Some scientists, for instance, want to understand the chemical mechanism behind acupuncture. To truly grasp it, however, researchers need to look at it from an energetic viewpoint, as the Chinese have been doing for thousands of years. Our Cartesian legacy makes us yearn for precise, definite answers. In a dynamic world full of natural phenomena that cannot be predicted nor measured, precise answers for every question are just not possible.

THE WHOLE OF IT

Traditional Chinese Medicine is not superior to the medicine of ancient Greeks. Hippocrates was not smarter or more sophisticated than Saint Hildegard. Descartes should be neither berated nor placed on a pedestal. And twenty-first-century quantum physics is not going to solve all the mysteries of medicine or disease. In other words, we gain nothing by favoring one era or one philosophy over another. Our ancestors from around the world have much to teach us. Learning from them requires respect for their diverse cultures and experiences, as well as discernment of their wisdom.

As alternative medicine grows in popularity, the rift becomes more prominent between those people eager to integrate the past into the present and those who are focused on our current medical model. Many alternative therapies, like acupuncture, homeopathy, and energy healing, came into being well before science discovered DNA helixes or began exploring cellular biology. Yet, the present tenets of science cannot explain how all of these therapies work.

Will there be a peaceful meeting of the minds? Will the Relman and Weil camps be able to synthesize and integrate their outlooks? Perhaps the late Thomas Kuhn, a professor at the Massachusetts Institute of Technology who coined the phrase "paradigm shift" in his classic book *The Structure of Scientific Revolutions,* understood what will eventually play out:

> Practicing in different worlds, the two groups of scientists see different things when they look from the same point in the same directions. Again, that is not to say that they can see anything they please. Both are looking at the world, and what they look at has not changed. But in some areas they see different things, and they see them in different relations one to the other. That is why a law that cannot even be demonstrated to one group of scientists may occasionally seem intuitively obvious to another. Equally, it is why, before they can hope to communicate fully, one group or the other must experience the conversion that we have been calling a paradigm shift.[6]

Well, I've decided not to wait around. By the time a paradigm shift gives the thumbs-up to alternative, integrative, and holistic medicine, or the gold standard of randomized, double-blind clinical trials validates homeopathy, herbal medicine, or visualization, my children will be grown up and taking care of themselves. I need remedies and philosophies that I can integrate into my life today. I want to know where the nearest emergency room is for setting a broken arm or stitching a cut, but I also want knowledge of home health care.

Most of us want to influence positively our children's health, well-being, and ultimate happiness. Just how do we accomplish such lofty goals? First, we judiciously embrace the ancient truths and practices that have assisted humankind in these endeavors for centuries. Second, we explore the role of spirituality in our lives. As one holistic doctor told me, health does not incorporate spirituality; spirituality embraces health—a concept we will address later. Finally, we give equal attention to our emotions, our minds, and our bodies. This is what being holistic is all about. It is the bright and the beautiful, the great and the small. The everything, the all.

It is the glory of life.

Let us experience it.

CHAPTER 4

Herbal Medicine: Relocating the Medicine Cabinet to the Kitchen

God makes the earth yield healing herbs
which the prudent man should not neglect.

SIRACH 38:4

The salt water washed against Gregg and me, soothing our jet-lagged bones as we and another couple body-surfed the ocean waves on our first day of a Caribbean vacation. Before Gregg could morph into a well-balanced amphibian, a mischievous wave playing linebacker plowed into his landlubber legs and pushed him across a bed of sand-camouflaged rocks, leaving him with an inch-long gash on the ball of his foot. Fortunately, the cut wasn't deep enough to warrant stitches.

Back at the house, Gregg scrounged up some antibacterial cream, which he applied for the next few days, but the cut remained obstinate. In fact, it rebelled by oozing and hurting more. When our friends Patricia and Steve departed a few days ahead of us, Steve, a medical doctor, left us with these parting words: "Lynn, watch that cut on Gregg's foot. If it gets worse or turns green, go see a doctor."

Great, I thought, a potential emergency right underfoot. The crisis brought to mind a remedy that I had learned about in Nepal but had never used. The recipe was simple: mix aloe vera gel and turmeric into a paste, apply it to the cut or scrape, and cover with a bandage. As it was, our Caribbean kitchen wasn't stocked with turmeric, and in my vacation inertia the antibacterial cream seemed safe and easy. So I had done nothing. Now I needed to act.

Fortunately, the British Virgin Island of Tortola is a spice haven, so we easily found turmeric at the local market. I cut a leaf from the backyard aloe clump, split it lengthwise, scooped out some gel with a spoon, sprinkled turmeric on it, and mixed the ingredients into a paste. I used the back of the spoon to spread the concoction onto Gregg's foot. The slight sting was nothing a piña colada couldn't cure. The next day, we were both amazed. The cut finally had dried and the skin was beginning to close over it.

I have since witnessed this simple remedy work its wonders many times. When my nephew burned the palm of his hand on a stove burner, I suggested aloe and turmeric. His neighbor, an emergency medical technician, was so impressed with how rapidly the wound healed that he asked what ointment had been used.

When my daughter wiped out on her bike, she suffered a nasty scrape on her side. She vehemently argued against any first aid beyond a bandage. Finally, in exasperation, I said, "So be it. Let's see what happens." A slight infection set in, which we nipped in the bud by smearing the aloe-turmeric potion over it. Within twenty-four hours, the healing process was in high gear.

A tube of commercially prepared, pure aloe gel and a small jar of turmeric are now standards in our traveling first aid kit, and our backyard boasts a clump of aloe. When my daughters get cuts, they like to mix the aloe and turmeric themselves. I just have to remind them to be careful: turmeric permanently stains fabric yellow!

HOLISTIC HERBALISM

Science now is confirming what I learned through experience: aloe and turmeric heals wounds. Aloe gel contains compounds that decrease inflammation, reduce pain, and promote healing of damaged tissue. Turmeric's constituents also are anti-inflammatory, antimicrobial, and analgesic. With more people clamoring for natural therapies, plant biochemistry, known as phytochemistry, is a hotbed of study. Researchers analyze plant components in order to learn how they influence the body.

Plants, however, are more than a cluster of individual compounds. Eliot Cowan's book *Plant Spirit Medicine: The Healing Power of Plants* tells about pharmaceutical company employees venturing into the depths of South American rain forests to meet with shamans, the resident medicine men who are well acquainted with the healing power of specific plants. The company people want to know which medicinal plants to harvest. They plan to study the plants' molecular structures, re-create them synthetically, patent them, and sell them to you and me. The shamans, says Cowan, just laugh.

Why do the shamans laugh? Because they view plants as living entities, pulsating with a life force all their own that can't be reproduced in a laboratory. When we use herbs, we tap into this energy. Dr. Julian Scott, a pediatrician trained in TCM, maintains the following in his book *Natural Medicine for Children:*

> Herbal medicine works on an energetic level, which recommends its use for babies and children. Their bodies are small and frail compared to adults, but their energy levels are much greater by far. As a result, the natural medicines, and particularly the herbal remedies, have striking and rapid effects.[1]

Who knows—maybe we all have felt the energy of plants but haven't been cognizant enough to identify it as such. Think about the plants and trees in and around your home or office, or in your favorite park, plaza, or promenade. Wouldn't those areas feel different without plants and trees? The spider plant and philodendra on my desk seem to greet me when I sit down to write. Maybe, as studies have shown, they respond to the music I play, though I can't tell if they prefer Beethoven or Neil Young. Some people believe that we need to ask a plant's permission to pick it or use it as medicine. Others, like shamans, believe that picking the plant without a prayer or ritual of blessing causes its medicines to remain in the soil.

One herbalist, in an introductory lecture on how to use herbs, had his novice audience meditate on a vase of calendula, also called pot marigold. "Feel the plant," he told them. "Let it talk. All you have to do is pay attention to the images and words that enter your mind." After ten minutes of silence, he asked them what they thought calendula could do medicinally. After listing all the answers, he discovered that the class had come up with the entire pharmacology of calendula, an herb that is used both externally, for burns, bruises, and other wounds, and internally, to induce perspiration and expel toxins through the skin.

You may buy into this theory of energy or you may slam-dunk it into the hocus-pocus trash can. Perhaps all we need do is acknowledge that plants are a part of nature and that by using them as medicine, we commune with nature. We get in step with the intricate, gyrating harmony that nature expresses every second of every millennium. When we create such a union, herbal medicine becomes something beyond a group of compounds that influences our health. It becomes one of the most natural, harmonious, and effective ways to heal and care for ourselves and our children.

HERBAL MEDICINE, PAST AND PRESENT

Modern-day America stems from a heritage rich in herbal medicine. Unfortunately, most of us are connected to this legacy by only a few withered grapevines hanging down the family tree. At one time, these vines were lush with remedies passed from generation to generation. Now we may learn about them through historical novels or movies, or perhaps we hear an elderly aunt reminisce about her great-grandmother's home remedies. When I learned how effectively our great-grandparents used herbal medicine, I felt the seeds of reverence sprout for the medicinal treasures we now are rediscovering.

Herbal medicine is thousands of years old. One of our more recent ancestors who promoted the home use of herbal medicine is the English apothecary Nicholas Culpeper (1616–1654). In his day, apothecaries were little more than doormats for doctors, a status that enraged Culpeper. He openly criticized the medical profession for hoarding its knowledge in Latin textbooks, which only the elite could read. Furthermore, he considered conventional medicines, particularly those containing mercury, to be harmful. The outspoken Culpeper bucked the trends and set up shop in a poor area of London, where he compassionately administered herbal remedies that healed many illnesses. While the local residents hailed him as an excellent physician, he became a stinging nettle to the medical doctors. Much to their alarm, he translated medical texts into English, dispersing the treasured information among his fellow apothecaries like dandelion seeds in the breeze. He then wrote *The English Physician,* an herbal book geared to the public. Even the uneducated, Culpeper believed, could learn to use the cornucopia of inexpensive, local herbs to heal themselves. He later expanded this book into *Culpeper's Complete Herbal: A Book of Natural Remedies for Ancient Ills.* Four hundred years later, the tome remains in print and is frequently referenced in herbal medicine books.

Culpeper reminds us that we can learn to safely and effectively use herbal remedies at home. Just think: we now have the opportunity to water the grapevines of herbal medicine, cultivate them, strengthen them, and keep them growing for future generations.

Safety First

Although the media often harps on herbal medicine's potential dangers, herbs remain relatively safe. Between 1981 and 1993, roughly 100,000 people in the United States died from adverse drug reactions, but no deaths during that time were attributable to commercial herb products.[11]

There are, however, legitimate safety issues concerning herbal medicine. First, beware of any botanical touted as a miracle cure-all. Of the thousands of herbs, many—like aloe—have a broad range of healing capabilities. Yet no single herb can cure every disease and disorder known to humankind. Nor can herbal supplements make up for diets lacking in proper nutrition. We still have to eat our spinach and brussels sprouts.

As we get acquainted with herbs, we sometimes make mistakes. We may think, for instance, that herbal medicines, because they are "natural," can be safely mixed with pharmaceutical medicines. The truth is, some combinations can be dangerous. Someone who takes Valium, a depressant, and then ingests valerian root, an herb containing sedative properties, may suffer serious problems. You should tell your medical doctor, homeopath, naturopath, Chinese-medicine practitioner, or whomever you see which herbal medicines you and your children use. If you or your child takes a prescription medicine and you wish to try an herbal remedy, consult a medical professional trained in herbal medicine.

Currently, herbs fall under the auspices of the Food and Drug Administration (FDA) and are regulated by the Dietary Supplement Health and Education Act, passed in October 1994. This legislation categorizes all herbal plant products as supplements, which gives consumers access to herbs. Of course, we want quality herbs that are not contaminated, mislabeled, or misidentified. Organizations like the American Botanical Council, the American Herbalist Guild, and the Herb Research Foundation are working with the FDA to create reasonable regulations that will ensure quality and availability.

If you are concerned about any of these issues, many people in the herb business can help you. I work with an herbalist who has owned an herb shop for twenty years. He knows which suppliers are reputable. He also knows how to use herbs, knows the potency of the various brands, and can recommend which herbs to use for specific ailments.

One final caution: If you or your child has a serious chronic illness, consult a professional who is well versed in herbal medicine. Treating acute conditions like fevers, sore throats, and nausea is much more straightforward than grappling with the complexities of diseases like arthritis, allergies, and attention deficit disorder.

Kitchen and Garden Remedies

Did you know that the odds are that you have an herbal medicine chest right in your spice cabinet, or growing in planters near your kitchen window, or just out the back door in your garden?

Rosemary, basil, parsley, and thyme are usually thought to be more culinary than medicinal, but they are extremely effective medicines. Not only is rosemary good in focaccia bread and on pork tenderloin, but, as Culpeper says, "It is a remedy for the windiness in the stomach, bowels, and spleen, and expels it powerfully."[2] In other words, it's an excellent digestive aid. Basil, a key ingredient in pesto, eases fever, cold, and flu symptoms when made into a tea. For thousands of years, parsley has been known as a diuretic, and thyme as an antiseptic. As you can see, your garden and spice cabinet are medicine chests.

At the end of this chapter, you will find a chart of common herbs and their medicinal uses. But first, we need to discuss how to buy these herbs (if you don't have a garden), store them, and prepare them. I can point you in the right direction so that when you or your child develops a cold or stomachache, you will be able to take some herbal action. Yet you have to take the initiative to jump off the diving board yourself. Fortunately, the plunge may be no deeper than an herbal bath containing a pint of chamomile tea.

No Garden? Buy in Bulk

If the rabbits go to town on your garden, or the kids' weekend softball schedule intrudes on your digging-in-the-dirt time, you can always buy herbs in bulk. Sometimes when I'm in a pinch, I buy jars of herbs at a local grocery store, but I prefer to buy herbs from a health food store or co-op. Not only can I buy them in bulk, I can find out if the herbs are organic, how fresh they are, and if they have undergone irradiation, a process that kills virulent microbes but is thought by many to damage foods. (More on food irradiation in chapter 7). Another advantage of buying bulk herbs is that they are considerably cheaper than herbs sold in jars. In addition, I can purchase a small amount of a spice I rarely use, like cayenne pepper, rather than a jar that will last two years.

Storing Herbs

If you grow your own herbs, you need to know which part of the plant to store, be it the flowers, seeds, leaves, or roots. If you buy in bulk, you purchase the herb in ready-to-use form. When I harvest garden herbs, such as oregano, I bunch the stems together and tie them at the bottom with a string, or loop a rubber band around them. I then hang the bunch upside down from a nail pounded into one of the kitchen walls. Dried in this position, the leaves are easier to strip from the stem. It's like aroma-art. Sometimes when I walk by I get a whiff of oregano; at other times, lemon balm or rosemary.

Not all plants dry at the same rate. Basil leaves are larger and take longer to dry than oregano leaves, for example—but most dry within five or six days. After the leaves dry, I strip them from the stem and put them in a glass jar in the spice cabinet. Since herbs lose their potency when exposed to light and oxygen, keep the jars in a cabinet rather than on the counter. I also store herbs bought in bulk in glass jars.

The rule of thumb is that herbs stay potent for about six months. If you properly store aromatic herbs, like rosemary and thyme, you can use them for over a year, particularly if they are homegrown and dried. Always smell the herb before using it; the intensity of its aroma is a good indication of its medicinal—as well as culinary—strength.

Herbal Preparations

Herbs can be prepared medicinally in a number of ways. Some concoctions are as simple as brewing tea, while others, like tonic wines, require more time and equipment. Since I'm short on the latter items, I tend to keep medicine-making really simple.

Infusions

An infusion is basically a strong tea, usually composed of 1 part herb to 20 parts water. This equals about 1 tablespoon per cup of water. Use half the amount of herbs when making an infusion for children. All you need is a stove burner for heating water, a tea kettle or pan, a container with a tight-fitting lid, and a strainer. Avoid aluminum and plastic cooking and storage containers, and please, please, don't make herbal remedies in the microwave. We'll talk about microwaves in more detail later; for now, know that if you can just adopt the no-microwave rule, your remedies will be that much more effective.

Infusions work best for leaves, flowers, and some stems. Use 1 teaspoon of dried herb per 1 cup of water. If the herbs are fresh, double that amount. Pour boiling water over the leaves, cover tightly, and let steep for ten to twenty minutes. I use a teapot with a tight-fitting lid, or place a saucer over a mug. Covering the infusion keeps the healing volatile oils released by the hot water from escaping. When the timer summons you, pour the tea through a strainer into a cup. You're ready to imbibe. If the tea is for your child, you may need to add a sweetener like pasteurized honey, brown rice syrup, stevia, or turbinado sugar (raw cane sugar). Avoid refined white sugar.

Extra infused tea can be refrigerated in a covered container for up to two days.

Decoctions

A decoction is relatively simple to make. It is best used for bark, roots, seeds, and some stems. Instead of steeping the herbs, you boil them, usually for twenty to thirty minutes. Use about 2 tablespoons of dried herb or 4 tablespoons of fresh herb to 3 cups of water. Again, use half the amount of herbs for children. The water will boil down to about 2 cups. Strain the resulting liquid, and drink. A decoction is stronger than an infusion—about 1 part herb to 10 parts water—but, like an infusion, can be stored in the refrigerator for two days. You may need to add a sweetener, especially for children.

When my husband was under the care of a TCM practitioner, he would come home with a brown paper bag full of intriguing barks and roots. In his case, he had to boil them in water for an hour, then drain off the muddy brown liquid. Most of the time, he managed to drink the tea without making a face. We Westerners want our medicines to taste tolerable, which can be a trick with certain herbs.

My favorite tasty decoction is made with ginger. I call it ginger tea, but technically it's a decoction. I peel about 2 inches of fresh gingerroot and boil it in 2 cups of water for a minimum of twenty minutes. The longer it boils, the stronger the tea. The kids prefer theirs with honey. Since ginger is an excellent digestive aid, it helps settle a rich meal—or any meal, for that matter. In addition, ginger tea soothes a sore throat, especially when made with honey or raw cane sugar, and it eases congestion, nausea, and motion sickness. Also, you can soak a washcloth in ginger tea and apply it to sore muscles for relief.

Once you start experimenting with herbs, you will soon find your favorite remedies.

Tinctures

A tincture, also called an extract, is stronger yet, being 1 part herb to 5 parts solvent. The solvent is usually composed of water plus at least 25 percent alcohol, which helps extract the plant's active ingredients and then preserves the mixture for up to two years. To be honest, I've never prepared a tincture; I buy mine at the health food store, although more and more drugstores carry them. Tinctures are usually sold in bottles of 1 fluid ounce that come with an eyedropper. The label indicates if the tincture is made with organic plants, and includes dosages.

As I write this, two bottles of children's echinacea tincture sit in our medicine cabinet. One is flavored orange and the other blackberry, and both use glycerin as a preservative, rather than alcohol. The flavoring does not alter the tincture's medicinal effectiveness. When my children have colds or get run down from busy schedules, I put the prescribed amount of drops in a glass and mix it with 2 to 4 ounces of juice. When I take echinacea, which I do when I'm feeling run down, stressed, or in the midst of a cold or other acute illness, I also use the children's tincture, mixed with water. Why buy the adult version when the children's is the same and tastes better?

Herbal Baths

Another very effective, but often overlooked, way of using herbs is in baths. Simply prepare 2 pints of a strong herbal infusion, strain, and add to a warm bath. For a fever, use tepid water. The warm water opens the skin's pores, which then absorb the volatile oils released in the infusion. The oils also enter the steam in the air. When inhaled through the mouth and nose, they enter the lungs and the bloodstream. An herbal bath allows the body to quickly assimilate the herb, sometimes faster than through the process of digestion. In addition, a warm bath soothes and relaxes. Soak in the bath for ten to thirty minutes. A child may be more willing to float in an herbal bath than drink herbal tea, particularly if the tea is bitter.

Other Preparations

Herbs can be used in many other forms, including poultices, compresses, capsules, suppositories, salves, lotions, eyewashes, and steam inhalations. An experienced herbalist can tell you which preparation is best for your particular need. Again, there are a number of good books that can instruct you on making these other preparations. Penelope Ody's *Home Herbal: A Practical Guide to Making Herbal Remedies for Common Ailments* even includes helpful photographs of how to make the medicines.

Dosages for You and Your Child

During acute illnesses, medicinal teas need to be taken in small doses frequently. A standard dosage for herbal tea (either an infusion or decoction) is three times a day. In her book *Herbal Remedies for Children's Health,* herbalist Rosemary Gladstar writes that for colds, fevers, and other acute ailments a child can take several small sips of tea every half hour until the symptoms abate. When my eight-year-old had a 100.2-degree fever, I gave her 2 tablespoons of sweetened basil tea every half hour. After three doses, her temperature was 98.9 degrees. I stopped the dosages, and within a few hours her temperature was back to normal.

Gladstar also suggests a mathematical formula to determine how much of an herbal medicine to administer to a child. First add 12 to the child's age. Then divide the child's age by this total. For my eight-year-old, I added 8 and 12 to get 20. Eight divided by 20 is .40. Thus, she needed a little less than half an adult dosage.[3]

Common Garden Herbs

Table 4.1 lists some common herbs that you can use to treat common acute ailments. You will find that more than one herb can be used to treat the same condition. Chamomile and dill, for instance, are both excellent colic remedies, and eight out of the ten herbs listed aid digestion. You may find that your body responds better to an infusion of chamomile than of dill. By experimenting, you'll learn which herbs best heal your body and your child's body.

I did not include the chemical properties of each plant. If you're curious about this area, you can consult many excellent books, some of which are listed in the recommended reading section at the back of this book. While research is still sorting out plant constituents and determining their roles in herbal medicines, the efficacy of the medicinal applications listed in Table 4.1 has been verified by practical use over hundreds of years. Used as an infusion, decoction, tincture, or herbal bath, these mild herbs are safe and effective.

TABLE 4.1

Herb	Plant Part Used	Preparation and Medicinal Use	Cautions
BASIL	Leaves	Standard infusion for: • Infant colic • Digestive aid • Fevers • Colds • Flu • Promotion of breast milk	Avoid essential oil during pregnancy
CATNIP (member of the mint family)	Leaves, flowers	Standard infusion for: • Fever reduction • Head colds • Flu • Infant colic • Stress reduction • Teething pain Tincture for: • Digestion (given before meals) • Calming fussy child (given before bed)	None
CHAMOMILE	Flowers (used in standard infusion), essential oil	Standard infusion for: • Infant colic (since chamomile passes through breast milk, mother should drink infusion)	Avoid essential oil during pregnancy

TABLE 4.1 (CONTINUED)

Herb	Plant Part Used	Preparation and Medicinal Use	Cautions
continued **CHAMOMILE**		• Teething pain • Digestive aid • Sedative, good for insomnia • Menstrual cramps (steep with two fresh ginger slices)	
DILL	Seeds	Standard infusion for: • Infant colic • Digestive aid • Expelling gas • Promoting flow of breast milk	None
LEMON BALM (also called Sweet Melissa; member of the mint family)	Leaves (fresh leaves best for medicinal uses)	Standard infusion for: • Viral inhibitor; (good for most acute childhood illnesses) • Mild sedative • Stress reduction • Digestive aid	None
PARSLEY	Leaves (rich in minerals and vitamin C)	Standard infusion for: • Diuretic • Promotes flow of breast milk • Digestive aid • Menstrual disorders	Avoid high leaf consumption during pregnancy or if you have kidney disease

Herb	Plant Part Used	Preparation and Medicinal Use	Cautions
RED RASPBERRY	Leaves, fruits (fruits are rich in vitamins and minerals, especially calcium and iron)	Standard infusion for: • Diarrhea and dysentery • Menstrual cramps; regulates heavy menstruation • Excellent uterine tonic during later pregnancy • Mouthwash for sore or infected gums	Avoid high doses of leaves during early pregnancy
ROSEMARY	Leaves	Standard infusion for: • Congestion, head and chest pain due to colds, allergies, or flu • Digestive aid • Hair rinse and baldness preventer Essential oil added to bath: • Stimulates mind and energy • Eases arthritis, rheumatism, and some headaches	Avoid essential oil during pregnancy

TABLE 4.1 (CONTINUED)

Herb	Plant Part Used	Preparation and Medicinal Use	Cautions
SAGE	Leaves	Standard infusion for: • Colds, fever, and flu • Digestive aid; expels gas • Sore throats and mouth ulcers (use as a gargle) • Soothes nerves and nervous conditions	Avoid high doses in pregnancy; do not use if epileptic
THYME	Leaves	Standard infusion for: • Respiratory ailments like colds, bronchitis, and whooping cough • Digestive aid • Nausea and diarrhea Essential oil for: • Wound care; good antiseptic (dilute and apply directly to wounds and infections under the skin)	Avoid high doses in pregnancy

CHAPTER 5

Homeopathy:
The Power of Nature

Homeopathy does not merely remove disease
from an organism; it strengthens and harmonizes
the very source of life and creativity in the individual.

GEORGE VITHOULKAS
THE SCIENCE OF HOMEOPATHY

The thermometer beeped and I quickly removed it from my five-year-old's mouth. Her temperature was 102.9 degrees. No wonder she was so flushed and listless at seven-thirty in the morning.

"Elle, honey, you have a fever. I'll get you a nice soft pillow and some remedies. You can rest here on the couch for a while, okay?" I said, rubbing her tummy, which felt much too warm.

As I headed for the medicine cabinet, I adjusted to the fact that I had to scratch my plans for the day. I scanned the bottles of homeopathic remedies that I had used to treat acute illnesses since Elle turned one year old. To this point, the stockpile of seven remedies, recommended by our family homeopath, had successfully treated fevers, vomiting, sore throats, earaches, coughs, runny and stuffy noses, and bruises.

I chose a bottle labeled "Ferrum phos." and tipped out two chalky white pills, slightly smaller in diameter than a pencil eraser. During Elle's last two bouts of fever, ferrum phosphoricum, or iron phosphate, had eased her symptoms. Every twenty minutes for the next two hours, Elle dissolved two of the sugary pills in her mouth. After the last dose, I rechecked her temperature. It registered 103.2 degrees—not good. I felt uneasy, as I always do when there is a fever in the house and a lump of a child on the couch. Because her fever wasn't alarmingly high, and less than half a day had passed, I felt no urgency to check in with our homeopath. Like a mother owl protecting the roost, however, I did feel a need to hover over the couch.

Something nagged me. Perhaps this fever had come on suddenly in the early morning hours, instead of gradually as I was assuming it had. I pulled out Dana Ullman's *Homeopathic Medicine for Children and Infants* and turned to the section on fever. It listed four remedies commonly used to treat varying types of fever: aconitum, arsonicum, belladonna, and ferrum phosphoricum. Choosing a remedy requires a close observation of symptoms. Is the child thirsty, pale, flushed, irritable, whiny, nervous, or restless? I have to remind myself to heed the emotional, as well as the physical, symptoms of an illness. This approach differs significantly from the allopathic approach, which recommends medicines like acetaminophen as a blanket treatment for all types of fever.

The book confirmed that ferrum phosphoricum is for a fever that comes on gradually. If the fever comes on suddenly, and the child is thirsty, restless, and easily chilled when uncovered, then aconitum is the remedy to try. But Elle wasn't restless. I knew belladonna was the remedy of choice after reading the following:

BELLADONNA: When children have a sudden onset of high fever with flushed faces and reddened lips, this remedy is the first to consider. These children also tend to have hot heads and cold extremities. The skin is usually so hot that it radiates heat (you can feel it by placing your hand a couple of inches away from the skin). The fever is a dry heat, without perspiration. The child tends to have a strong and bounding pulse. At night the temperature gets its highest, making the child agitated, sometimes delirious, perhaps leading her to hallucinate.[1]

From *Homeopathic Medicine For Children and Infants* by Dana Ullman, coyright © 1992 by Dana Ullman. Used by permission of Jeremy P. Tarcher, a division of Penguin Putnam Inc.

We never had needed this remedy before, so I hustled to the health food store to buy some belladonna 6x. Back at home, I resumed the same routine: two pills every twenty minutes. After an hour, the thermometer read 100.2 degrees. Ahhh, relief. By the end of the day, her temperature was normal, and by the next afternoon, she was chasing a soccer ball around the yard. Not a bad recovery rate, considering that the malady laid up many of her peers or their parents for a week.

HOMEOPATHY, PAST TO PRESENT

Although medical textbooks from ancient China, India, and Greece refer to homeopathic concepts, the science as it is now practiced originated about two hundred years ago with the German physician Samuel Hahnemann (1755–1843). Hahnemann not only pursued a career as a physician, but was also a respected chemist and was fluent in at least eight languages. When Hahnemann started practicing medicine, common treatments included bloodletting, the administration of toxic medicinals to induce vomiting and purge the bowels, and the application of hot substances on the skin to draw out infection, a technique called blistering. This protocol quickly disillusioned Hahnemann. For him, these fierce treatments violated the Hippocratic maxim "First, do no harm." He began writing articles critical of the medical establishment and espousing a proper diet, personal hygiene, fresh air, and exercise. A prolific writer, Hahnemann garnered much attention—and respect—as a result of his many published articles.

While a professor of medicine at Leipzig University in Germany, he started translating medical texts into German. He was working on a book written by the Scottish physician William Cullen when a curious comment caught his attention. Cullen claimed that quinine, which is extracted from the bark of the Peruvian cinchona tree, cures malaria because of its bitter and astringent properties. With his strong background in chemistry, Hahnemann knew of other, more astringent substances that had no effect on malaria.

Hahnemann then wondered what cinchona would do to a healthy person. If it cured a person of malaria, could it induce malaria-like symptoms in a healthy person? He decided to test this theory by ingesting large doses of cinchona, after which he did indeed develop symptoms similar to those of malaria, including fever and chills. When he stopped the cinchona doses, the symptoms disappeared. If a large dose of medicine could induce symptoms in a healthy person, he reasoned, perhaps a small amount might eliminate them in an ill person. Through much chemical experimentation, Hahnemann created a technique he called potentization.

Basically, he took 1 part of a medicinal plant, like cinchona, and diluted it with 99 parts of distilled water or ethyl alcohol. Then he took 1 part of that mixture and again diluted it with 99 parts of distilled water or ethyl alcohol. He repeated this process over and over. Between dilutions, he added kinetic energy to the solution by shaking it, a process he named succussion. The remedies were not effective unless they were both diluted and succussed. Once he began using these remedies as treatment, Hahnemann discovered that the more diluted the medicine, the more therapeutic it was.

He called this concept of "like curing like" the "Law of Similars." When I gave my daughter belladonna, I actually gave her a dilution of a poisonous plant known as deadly nightshade. In its crude form, deadly nightshade is, indeed, deadly. Similarly, the remedy Rhus toxicodendron (Rhus tox.), which is diluted poison ivy, cures poison ivy rash and itching. Ipecacuanha (Ipec.) is diluted ipecac root. Poison control centers recommend using ipecac to induce vomiting in children if they swallow a poisonous substance; in its homeopathic form, ipecac helps stop vomiting.

The medical community thought Hahnemann had flipped his lid. How could such infinitesimal amounts of medicine cure anything? his opponents wondered. While his colleagues called him a quack and a charlatan, stories spread among the public of homeopathy's success in treating scarlet fever, cholera, skin disorders, and a myriad of other diseases. Hahnemann's practice flourished and his fame spread across Europe and overseas. By the end of his life, in spite of conventional medicine's continued skepticism, he had a strong following of doctors, medical students, and laypeople.

After Hahnemann's death, homeopathy's popularity continued in Europe and the United States. Many famous people have supported the medicine, including John D. Rockefeller, who lived to age ninety-nine; Mahatma Gandhi; and England's royal family, who continues to use it. Even Mary Baker Eddy, the founder of Christian Science, approved of homeopathy.

The American Medical Association (AMA), however, has always been reluctant to recognize the science and practice of homeopathy. From the beginning, homeopathy threatened conventional medicine with its popularity, low cost, and ease of application. Founded in 1846 as a rival to the American Institute of Homeopathy, which had formed two years earlier, the AMA gained the legislative upper hand. The AMA considered homeopathy to be quackery, and for a period of time would not allow its members to practice it. The AMA's influence became apparent by the 1920s. At the turn of the century,

America boasted 22 homeopathic schools, 29 homeopathic medical journals, 100 homeopathic hospitals, and 1,000 homeopathic pharmacies. By 1923 only two schools of homeopathy remained open.[2]

Yet no institution or person has succeeded in snuffing out the practice of homeopathy. In fact, the United States is now experiencing a resurgence of devotees. Sales of homeopathic remedies in 1996 amounted to $227 million, and they continue to increase by at least 12 percent per year.[3] An estimated six million Americans use homeopathy.[4] Interestingly, the use of homeopathy in other countries is far more widespread. In France, 70 percent of physicians view homeopathy favorably and the national health care system reimburses the cost of remedies.[5] The Danish government recently accepted homeopathy as a standard form of medicine. It is also used extensively in Sweden, Germany, Italy, Britain, eastern Europe, South America (particularly Argentina and Brazil), and India. Over 120 four- and five-year homeopathic schools operate in India. In Bombay, the Homeopathy India Foundation runs two clinics, the Sanjivak Center and the Life Force Clinic, which each treat thirty to forty patients a day exclusively with homeopathy. Patients' illnesses run the gamut from acute conditions like tonsillitis, pneumonia, and food poisoning to chronic conditions like migraines, rheumatoid arthritis, and asthma.

BELIEVERS AND NONBELIEVERS

I became hooked on homeopathy after a harrowing Wisconsin winter during which Gregg, the kids, and I moved from one acute illness to another. I resolved to learn a few basics of homeopathy. Before the first frost of the next fall, I attended a lecture that focused on four or five remedies for flus, colds, sore throats, and earaches. The following winter, we totaled no more than four or five sick days among us. The remedies we used are listed in the chart at the end of this chapter.

Those of us who rely on homeopathy usually have little need for an antibiotic during acute illnesses. Homeopathy is especially good for children, for a number of reasons. Remedies are easy to take; in pill form, they taste like sugar and dissolve in one's mouth. You can buy remedies at most health food stores and an increasing number of mainstream pharmacies. They are relatively inexpensive—I paid about $8.00 for 100 belladonna tablets, which will never expire, and Elle needed no more than ten tablets. Finally, those of us who use homeopathic remedies know that they work quickly, and with no side effects, when used in the recommended dosages.

Why, if advocates just about stake their lives on it, does homeopathy remain so controversial within the medical arena? The science that supports conventional medicine has trouble opening its arms to homeopathy because the language that this science uses to explain chemical reactions and cell metabolism cannot explain homeopathy. The primary reason for this communication gap is that most remedies do not contain even one molecule of the substance used. The question raised during Hahnemann's time persists: How can a medicine that contains no molecules of its active ingredient possibly affect the body?

According to the principles established by the nineteenth-century chemist Amedeo Avogadro, solutions diluted beyond a certain point do not contain any molecules of the original substance. Hahnemann diluted his solutions by either one-tenth or one-one hundredth. Those diluted by one-tenth are denoted by the letter x, the Roman numeral for ten. Likewise, solutions diluted by one-one hundredth are denoted by the letter c, the Roman numeral for 100. According to Avogadro's law, solutions diluted beyond 12c or 24x, which are roughly equivalent dilutions, do not contain any molecules of medicine. Ironically, the more diluted the remedy, the stronger it is. Homeopaths speculate that the energy, or the resonance, of a substance is transferred to water during the dilution and succussion process. This energy then influences the body. Homeopathy is often called ultramolecular medicine or energy medicine.

Because of this seemingly bizarre theory, articles, books, and scientists decry homeopathy as an impossible and worthless form of medicine. It is a medicine that contradicts the basic laws of chemistry and physics. Nonbelievers contend that homeopathy "cannot possibly produce any effect" because of the infinite dilution of the agents used.[6] One skeptic even calls the science of homeopathy "a pernicious form of paraherbalism."[7]

But between these sharp blades of doubt, support for homeopathy grows. An increasing number of scientific studies accompany this growth.

STUDIES SUPPORTING HOMEOPATHY

Research shows that homeopathy effectively treats acute and chronic conditions. In a 1996 study originally published in German, parents of 131 children chose either homeopathic or conventional care for acute otitis media. One hundred three children took homeopathic remedies, and 28 took antibiotics. In the homeopathic group, the recurrence of ear infections was .41 per patient, and of this group suffering repeat infections, 29.3 percent had a maximum of three recurrences. The children treated with antibiotics had an ear infection recurrence of .70 per patient and of those patients with more than one infection, 43.5 percent had a maximum of six recurrences.[8]

The first homeopathic study published in America, in the May 1994 issue of *Pediatrics,* reviewed the treatment of acute childhood diarrhea with homeopathic medicine. Eighty-one Nicaraguan children between the ages of six months and five years received remedies individualized to each child's symptoms. The group receiving remedies experienced a 20 percent faster cure rate than the group given the placebo.[9]

British scientists conducted two of the largest studies on homeopathy. The first, an analysis of research conducted over twenty-five years, called a meta-analysis, was published in 1991 in the *British Medical Journal*. The researchers examined 107 controlled trials of homeopathy and deemed 22 of them to be of high caliber. Much to the surprise of the research team, 15 of these higher-caliber trials showed homeopathy to be effective.[10] An even more significant meta-analysis was published in the *Lancet* in 1997. This time, 89 trials were studied. The researchers concluded that the results were "not compatible with the hypothesis that the clinical effects of homeopathy are completely due to placebo." Although they cautiously suggested that evidence was insufficient to label homeopathy as "clearly efficacious in treating any single clinical condition," they encouraged further research on homeopathy.[11]

A study published in the *British Homeopathic Journal* in 1997 focused on attention deficit hyperactivity disorder (ADHD). Forty-three children diagnosed with ADHD were randomly assigned to either a placebo or a homeopathic remedy. In keeping with the practice of homeopathy, the remedies were designed for each child, depending on their specific symptoms. Results clearly indicated that those children taking remedies experienced significant improvement.

Homeopaths Judyth Reichenberg-Ullman and Robert Ullman describe their success in treating children with attention deficit disorder (ADD) in their book *Ritalin-Free Kids: Safe and Effective Homeopathic Treatment of ADD and Other Behavioral and Learning Problems*. They have found that homeopathy helps about 70 percent of patients. Sometimes symptoms improve noticeably within a few days or weeks; sometimes treatment must continue for at least a year for a child to experience long-term benefits.[12] Roughly four and a half million children in the United States are diagnosed with ADD, of whom more than two million take Ritalin or other stimulants that have documented side effects. This is five times the amount of pharmaceuticals prescribed for children in all other countries combined. Homeopathy, which has no side effects, is worthy of serious consideration by parents and researchers alike.

Skeptics contend that homeopathic remedies amount to nothing more than placebos, but homeopathy is used successfully in treating infants and animals. Does a baby know that a sweet-tasting homeopathic remedy is medicine? Does an infant even know what medicine is? Likewise, does a horse know that a homeopathic remedy will help heal a malady? Of course not. The Academy of Veterinary Homeopathy promotes homeopathy as a treatment for illness in large and small animals.

EXPERIENCE AS PROOF

If homeopathy sounds intriguing, you have two options. You can stock up on patience for a few decades, or maybe a century or two, and wait until our medical science salutes homeopathy as a valid healing method. Or you can just give it a try. You may feel more comfortable trying remedies if you have a bit more understanding of the philosophy behind the medicine, so read on.

Vital Energy

Driving the body's health is what homeopaths often call the vital force, which is synonymous with vital energy. In Chinese medicine, this energy is called chi. (See chapter 3 for a discussion of *chi*.) Basically, it is the dynamic energy system that resonates within the human body. In his book *The Science of Homeopathy*, George Vithoulkas describes it this way:

The vital force is an influence that directs all aspects of life in the organism. It adapts to environmental influences, it animates the emotional life of the individual, it provides thoughts and creativity, and it conducts spiritual inspiration.[13]

The body's immune system, cellular biology, and even its DNA are manifestations of this vital energy. Most of us don't pay attention to or feel these resonating energies. We go about our morning routine of packing lunches for our kids, helping them find their shoes, and kissing and hugging them good-bye. All the while, our vital energy integrates the many events that affect our physical, psychological, mental, and spiritual beings. "Every stimulus, every emotion, and every thought has a corresponding effect to some degree on all levels of the body simultaneously and instantaneously," writes Vithoulkas. Our immune systems, for instance, integrate many stimuli: viruses, bacteria, chemicals, and even something as simple as a cold draft. If this system is not strong enough to accomplish this integration, due to hereditary weakness or a very strong stimulus, then we may become ill. Our bodies, previously at ease, now experience *dis*-ease.

Although the exact mechanism of homeopathic remedies has not yet been clearly defined, the theory is that remedies act on an energetic level. They help balance our vital energy. When this energy moves freely throughout our bodies, our organs and systems operate efficiently and disease remains absent.

The Body's Innate Intelligence

Another principle integral to homeopathy concerns the body's innate intelligence. Every single human cell knows how to respond in the most appropriate way at any given moment. Thus, our tissues, organs, and systems—along with our emotions, mind, and spirit—

constantly strive to create or maintain health. The body instinctively swings toward homeostasis or balance.

I have a tendency to forget this fact. When my nose becomes a faucet, I'm usually not in the mood to applaud my body's ability to discharge toxins. When my daughter's cough accompanies the coyotes' howls in the wee hours of the morn, I don't sing, "Hallelujah, she's strengthening her respiratory system." When they first appear, these acute symptoms irritate me. I have learned, however, to remind myself that they signify healing. Hence, a quick fix is not necessarily in my or my child's best interest. A fever, for example, indicates that the immune system is alert and on the job and creating an unpleasant environment for bacteria and viruses. I don't suppress the fever, because that would only prolong the illness.

My friend Caroline told me one day that her daughter had missed preschool the day before due to a fever. She said that shortly after she had given Hayley some acetaminophen, the four-year-old was running around and playing. Four hours later, Hayley was slumped in bed again, feverish. The healing process automatically resumes when given the opportunity to do so.

The fact that the body takes care of itself doesn't mean that I won't support it during the healing process. Homeopathy, herbs, and diet are a few of the natural ways to encourage healing. Because homeopathic remedies work on an energetic level, they do not drive illness deeper into the body, nor do they have side effects. Chemical drugs, on the other hand, are not designed to work this way; they affect the body differently, sometimes generating side effects, which signify an imbalance in the body. Have you ever seen someone go on antibiotics for a sinus infection, only to develop bronchitis a few months later, take stronger antibiotics, and, at some point down the road, after an on-again, off-again stint with various prescriptions, develop asthma? Antibiotics may hinder the body's ability to completely heal itself, whereas homeopathy does not barricade the body's innate healing process.

Individuality

Although allopathy and homeopathy both treat disease according to symptoms, the two differ significantly. Homeopathy focuses on the individual. Even though you and I share characteristics, I am very different from you. My patterns of living differ. My tastes differ. I feel and see the world in my own unique way. If we get a cold at the same time, we may need different remedies since our bodies go about reestablishing balance in different ways.

One summer my daughter and I returned from vacation with ear infections. Had we seen a conventional doctor, we may very well have ended up with the same antibiotic even though our symptoms differed. Her ear ached and she had a stuffy nose with yellow discharge; my ear, which was not in pain, felt as if I had overextended my stay in an airplane's pressurized cabin, and I had a runny nose with white discharge. We needed different remedies. She took silicea 6x and I took kali muriaticum (Kali mur.) 6x, and we both recovered within a few days.

THE PRACTITIONER: THE HOMEOPATH

During a consultation, a homeopath will take into account your total being, which includes everything about you: the spiritual, emotional, mental, and physical. Since these four levels constantly interact and influence each other, to consider anything less would lead to an incomplete diagnosis and, possibly, an inappropriate treatment. The entire body participates in disease and the restoration of balance; therefore, every symptom is pertinent. A homeopath will inquire about your aches, pains, and disorders, but also will ask about your diet, family medical history, sleep habits, work habits, emotional state, and so on.

Because homeopathy treats the entire person, it does not require specialists. A homeopath who treats a patient with asthma will continue to treat that patient if his symptoms change to ones of anxiety. These conditions are interrelated. In fact, homeopaths concur that almost no disease exists without involving our emotional level. You can observe this phenomenon in children. I remember one night when my daughter threw herself on the floor in an uncharacteristic crying fit. The next day, she awoke with a slight fever. Sometimes illness begins with an emotional imbalance, other times with a physical imbalance.

Although homeopathy is a science based on principles, art comes into play during treatment. A homeopath chooses a remedy that will influence particular life processes. All homeopaths use a *materia medica*. This is a book that lists individual remedies and alone with specific symptoms that each remedy targets. Sometimes the symptoms for a remedy are quite diverse. Chamomilla (chamomile), for instance, can be used for symptoms of earache, teething, colic, insomnia, and upset stomach.

At first glance, you may think that all you need to do is acquire a materia medica and start trying out remedies. Ear infections and colds are acute situations that you and I, as laypeople, can learn to handle with some professional guidance. For long-term care, however, consult a trained homeopath who knows how to assess your individual constitution, who understands how the remedies affect the energetic levels of the body, and who has been trained in how different remedies interact with each other.

Some homeopaths work in the classical tradition established by Hahnemann. This means that no more than one remedy is used at a time. Other homeopaths combine remedies. Similarly, one homeopath may use high-potency remedies while another may rely on low-potency ones. I'm accustomed to working with a professional who may suggest three or four remedies, but generally in low doses.

REMEDIES: A SIMPLE STARTING POINT

The golden rule I learned for the home use of remedies is to keep it simple. Learning to use a few remedies effectively is the best way to initiate yourself into the practice of homeopathy. I primarily use low doses of tissue salts, also called cell salts. These are minerals, like calcium phosphate and sodium chloride, that are naturally found in human cells. There are twelve cell salts, and all are essential for organs and tissues to function properly. If the molecular action of the body's cell salts becomes disturbed, disease may result. Potentized cell salts, also called tissue remedies, help restore equilibrium to the body's cell salts. I purchase tissue remedies in the 6x potency; if that potency is unavailable, I buy the 12x potency.

In addition, I have used remedies that are not tissue salts, such as belladonna 6x. I keep Apis mellifica 6LM on hand for bee stings and other insect bites where there is swelling, burning, or stinging pains. (*LM* is a much higher potency than *x*. Use no more than two doses within a fifteen-minute interval. If the remedy is correct, it should start working almost immediately.) Arnica montana (arnica) 30c is in our medicine cabinet for bumps and bruises. As Dana Ullman says, arnica is the "aspirin of homeopathy for injuries."[14]

Most remedies are sold individually, but combination remedies for maladies including sore throats, colds, and allergies are also available. I have had better results with the individual remedies. When I get a sore throat, Ferrum phos. works better for me than a combination remedy sold for sore throats. The one combination remedy worth trying is Hyland's Teething Tablets. This low-dose combination remedy includes chamomilla 3x. The label includes dosages for infants and children.

If you are hesitant to try remedies on your own, find a homeopath who can guide you through a few acute illnesses. As you develop a feel for how remedies work, your confidence will increase and you may find that you require outside guidance less and less. Remember that the body, for whatever reason, may need to progress through all the stages of a cold or flu, even when homeopathic remedies are used. My experience in such a case is that the overall duration of the illness tends to be shorter, even when it includes all the stages.

Dosages

- Use 6x potency in tablet form rather than liquid form. Liquid remedies contain alcohol, which may aggravate a child.
- Follow the dosage direction on the bottle. Give children half of an adult dosage.
- When giving remedies to infants, crush the tablets with a plastic spoon. A metal spoon can interfere with the remedy's action. Mix the powdered remedy with a teaspoon of breast milk or a teaspoon of water and place in the infant's mouth.
- During acute symptoms, administer tablets every fifteen minutes, but after six dosages change to every hour. If nothing has changed after the first hour following the six dosages, you may need to change remedies.
- Always observe the symptoms. Three things can happen:
  1. The symptoms stay the same. In this case, administer the remedy three times a day for one or two days. If no change occurs, you may need to try a different remedy.
  2. The symptoms improve or resolve themselves. If the symptoms resolve themselves and end, stop administering remedies. If the symptoms improve, start cutting back in

TABLE 5.1

Simple Guide to Using Tissue Remedies

Symptom	Remedy
Early stages of illness including irritability, low energy, lack of appetite, fussiness, and whining	Ferrum phos.
Fever • First stages of all fevers • High fevers	 Ferrum phos. Ferrum phos.
Phlegm and/or exportation from ears, nose, and throat • Clear • Whitish • Yellow or yellow-green	 • Ferrum phos. • Kali. mur. • Kali. sulph., Natrum sulph., and Silicea If high fever is present, also give Ferrum phos.
Sore throat (Remember to look in the throat!) • Red, inflamed throat • Whitish spots on tonsils • Swollen glands, painful throat, pain when swallowing	 • Ferrum phos. • Kali. phos. • Calc. phos.
Nausea and/or vomiting	• Mag. phos.
Loose bowels and/or diarrhea • Watery stools • Greenish stools • Yellowish stools	 • Kali phos. • Natrum sulph. • Kali sulph.
Earaches • Whitish coating on tongue • Sharp, stitching pain • Swollen glands	 • Kali. mur. • Ferrum phos. • Kali. mur. and Calc. phos.
Restitution and recovery • Acute symptoms are gone, but low energy, weakness, paleness, and so on remain.	 • Kali. phos. and Calc. sulph. Give three times a day for up to a week.

Note: The only two tissue salts that should not be used simultaneously are Calc. sulph. and silicea.

dosages. Give the remedy two times per day until symptoms resolve. If symptoms change to different symptoms, give a new remedy.

3. The symptoms change. In this case, match the new symptom to a remedy.

- HELPFUL HINT: Ferrum phos. is the best remedy to give at the first sign of illness, because it often initiates the healing process before acute or serious symptoms develop. If you observe, for instance, that your child (or significant other) is fussy, whining, nervous, irritable, listless, overtired, or not hungry, try giving her Ferrum phos. three times a day for two or three days. Even if the child is simply overtired, the remedy will not harm her and should help restore balance.

- If symptoms are serious, such as a prolonged high fever or fluid in the lungs, consult a professional homeopath or other health care practitioner.

CHAPTER 6

Ayurveda: 5,000 Years Old and Still Healthy

*The voyage of discovery lies not in seeking new vistas
but in having new eyes.*

—WILLIAM BUTLER YEATS

In 1994 I began a two-week seminar in Kathmandu, Nepal, on Ayurveda (pronounced "eye-er-VAY-da"), the Eastern Indian system of health and medicine. Although I knew well in advance what aspects of Ayurveda the lectures would cover, the only part of the course outline that I could think about was the lecture on how to use spices and herbs during illness. I was eager to gather these nuggets of knowledge right away. Perhaps they would make the inevitable acute maladies of life—particularly those of childhood—easier for patient and caregiver to endure.

On the first day of class, disappointment shook me awake. The instructor reminded us that the philosophy of Ayurveda would precede its practical applications. So the class plowed through a week of the theory behind the practice, just as you have to plow through my research. By the time I learned that ginger alleviates stomach cramps and coriander eases nausea, I was no longer seeing herbs and spices as merely "natural" medicines for acute illness. They were medicines, all right, but I now saw them in relation to a science that has precisely and logically addressed health and disease for an estimated five thousand years.

Ayurveda probably has influenced my view of life more than any other philosophy. For me, it explains much of the world. Within its framework, I have come to understand, as you will, too, how I am able to clean up the breakfast mess, start the laundry, and possibly squeeze in a few other chores while my children s-l-o-w-l-y pick out their clothes and put them on, brush their teeth, and tie their shoes. Ayurveda elucidates my daughter's emotional and gregarious nature. Ayurveda explains my sweet tooth, my discomfort in Arizona's summer heat, and my flare-ups of anger when I'm too hungry. If I sleep until 9:00 A.M. instead of rising at dawn, I know why I'm sluggish all day despite the extra hours of rest. I also know why spicy foods throw off my digestion during times of stress. I see why some people tolerate caffeine, while others don't. Ayurveda enlightens me and guides me in the choices I make in living my life, and it lends a deeper understanding to the events and patterns around me.

Ayurveda is a philosophy that embodies many practical suggestions for creating good health on all levels. Anyone who is familiar with Ayurveda will verify that it is an intricate science, particularly when used by Ayurvedic doctors. However, you need only learn some of the basics of Ayurveda in order to apply it skillfully on a daily basis. Although this chapter covers just a few basics, you may find that these morsels of insight shine like little beacons on our mysterious, shadowed world.

ORIGINS

Sometime between three and five thousand years ago in India, the Hindu holy books known as the *Vedas* were created. The Vedas actually are a compilation of ancient writings that include religious texts as well as texts on health. The authors of these classical writings were called *rishis*. "Rishi" is a title for a person who lives a contemplative life and intently studies the laws of nature and of humankind. The Vedas present the wisdom of the rishis in timeless, poetic writings.

A portion of the Vedas addresses the science of daily living. In Sanskrit, the rishis' native language, this science is called Ayurveda. *Ayur* means "life cycle" or "daily life" and *veda* means "wisdom." Thus, Ayurveda is the wisdom of life. Being a holistic philosophy, it explains the relationships among the body, mind, and spirit. Ayurveda also includes a very intricate medical system that addresses pediatrics, gynecology and obstetrics, toxicology, ophthalmology, otolaryngology, general medicine, general surgery, and geriatrics. Doctors of Ayurveda, the majority of whom are found in India and Nepal, rigorously study and train in Ayurvedic medicine for at least five years. Although comprehensive and complex, Ayurveda also provides the layperson with simple tools for self-care and self-healing.

THE BASICS: RELATIONSHIPS AND QUALITIES

One doesn't usually broach the topic of health with a discussion of relationships, but for our purposes it's a good starting point. When we think of relationships, we are inclined to think of how we interact with people. Some people, for example, make us feel sunny and light while others drag us down into the dark dumps. Consider your interpersonal relationships for a moment. In my case, I have a unique relationship with my husband and with each of my daughters. These relationships differ from the ones that I have with my parents, siblings, long-time friends, and neighbors.

Bear in mind that relationships extend beyond the sea of humanity. In fact, relationships exist among everything imaginable. The crunchy apple in the fruit drawer, the prickly pear cactus in the backyard, the Arizona sun, and the moon all draw me into a relationship. To tell you the truth, I don't give much thought to some of these relationships. I'm not aware that a full moon affects me any differently than a new moon. I know the seasons make me feel different; my skin is much dryer in winter than during the humid summer. Likewise, an apple sometimes jump-starts my brain, so I can't help but gobble it; other times, it makes me feel cold, so I toss it out half eaten. You see, relationships are never static. Every day and every moment, they shift and change.

At the heart of relationships are qualities. Everyone and everything has multiple qualities. When one quality interacts with another, a relationship forms. Think of a person with whom you would enjoy spending morning, noon, and night. What qualities do you love in that person? His humor, compassion, empathy, adventurous spirit, perseverance, or appearance? Now think of a person with whom you wouldn't even want to share a cappuccino. What qualities does that person exude?

Now, once again, think beyond people. That crunchy, airy apple in the fruit drawer has different qualities from a hamburger. Each of these foods probably affects you differently. You may feel energized after eating an apple and a bit sedentary after eating a hamburger. Most likely, you respond to the qualities of seasons differently. The cooler air of early winter may refresh you more than the heat of midsummer. Even diseases have qualities. Chicken pox is red, hot, and itchy, while a cold is watery and runny or, perhaps, stuffy and immobile.

When our qualities interact with the qualities of other people or things, particular relationships develop. In essence, Ayurveda explains how these relationships influence the body, mind, and spirit.

Seeing the relationships among your qualities and the qualities of all around you will give you more insight into the workings of the world. As I hope you realize by now, such a vision doesn't develop overnight. You're not going to say, "Hey, cool, after reading one chapter on Ayurveda, the world makes so much more sense." But if you learn a few basics of Ayurveda—that is, a few things about relationships and qualities—and apply those basics to the events around you, you will begin to recognize which relationships are healthiest for you. A relationship with ginger tea, for instance, might be healthier than a relationship with coffee. You won't even need a Ph.D. in biochemistry to figure out why. What's more, you will be able to identify the relationships that are best for your children. As a result, you can create and foster those healthy relationships.

Now that's cool.

THE DOSHAS

Ayurveda groups qualities into categories called *doshas* (pronounced DOH-shas). Doshas aren't something physical that you can touch or measure. Rather, doshas are tools for classifying by qualities everything around us. They create a point of reference from which we can judge and understand the complexities of our world. The three main doshas are *vata, pitta,* and *kapha.*

Like any science, Ayurveda has its own language. Initially, some of these words may stick to your tongue, but don't worry: this chapter only dishes out a handful of vocabulary. Of all these terms, the three most important to remember are vata, pitta, and kapha.

Most people have all three doshas in their being, also called a constitution. Generally, however, one or two doshas dominate a person's constitution. When our doshas become imbalanced, disease can occur. For any type of self-healing to transpire, it is helpful to know the roles that vata, pitta, and kapha play in our bodies, our emotions, our spirits, and even our environment.

Before we get into a discussion of the doshas, take a minute to complete the questionnaire on the next page (Table 6.1) in order to determine your doshic constitution. Almost every book on Ayurveda contains a variation of this questionnaire. When I bought my first book about Ayurveda, *Perfect Health: The Complete Mind/Body Guide* by Deepak Chopra, I didn't know anything about Ayurvedic philosophy, and I certainly had no comprehension of doshas. (You may be in the same position now.) At that time, the idea of classifying people according to three categories seemed hokey, like a bad version of astrology where you find yourself described under more than one zodiac sign. Now that I have a deeper understanding of Ayurveda, I realize how carefully and accurately doshas explain the qualities of people, plants, animals, food, weather, and all else around us, including the events that continuously occur in our dynamic world.

TABLE 6.1

The Human Constitution *(Prakruti)*

Aspect of Constitution	Vata	Pitta	Kapha
☐ Frame	Thin	Moderate	Thick
☐ Body Weight	Low	Moderate	Overweight
☐ Skin	Dry, Rough, Cool, Brown, Black	Soft, Oily, Warm, Fair, Red, Yellowish	Thick, Oily, Cool, Pale, White
☐ Hair	Black, Dry, Kinky	Soft, Oily, Yellow, Early Gray, Red	Thick, Oily, Wavy, Dark or Light
☐ Teeth	Protruded, Big and Crooked, Gums Emaciated	Moderate in Size, Soft Gums, Yellowish	Strong, White
☐ Eyes	Small, Dull, Dry, Brown, Black	Sharp, Penetrating, Green, Gray, Yellow	Big, Attractive, Blue, Thick Eyelashes
☐ Appetite	Variable, Scanty	Good, Excessive, Unbearable	Slow but Steady
☐ Taste	Sweet, Sour, Saline	Sweet, Bitter, Astringent	Pungent, Bitter, Astringent
☐ Thirst	Variable	Excessive	Scanty
☐ Elimination	Dry, Hard, Constipated	Soft, Oily, Loose	Thick, Oily, Heavy, Slow
☐ Physical Activity	Very Active	Moderate	Lethargic
☐ Mind	Restless, Active	Aggressive, Intelligent	Calm, Slow

TABLE 6.1 (continued)

Aspect of Constitution	Vata	Pitta	Kapha
☐ Emotional Temperament	Fearful, Insecure, Unpredictable	Aggressive, Irritable, Jealous	Calm, Greedy, Attached
☐ Faith	Changeable	Fanatic	Steady
☐ Memory	Recent Memory Good, Remote Memory Poor	Sharp	Slow but Prolonged
☐ Dreams	Fearful, Flying, Jumping, Running	Fiery, Anger, Violence, War	Watery, River, Ocean, Lake, Swimming, Romantic
☐ Sleep	Scanty, Interrupted	Little but Sound	Heavy, Prolonged
☐ Speech	Fast	Sharp and Cutting	Slow, Monotonous
☐ Financial Status	Poor, Spends Money Quickly on Trifles	Moderate, Spends on Luxuries	Rich, Moneysaver, Spends on Food
☐ Pulse	Thready, Feeble, Moves Like a Snake	Moderate, Jumping Like a Frog	Broad, Slow, Moves Like a Swan

NOTE: Circles have been provided next to the aspects for those who wish to determine a general idea of individual constitutional make-up. Mark *V* for Vata, *P* for Pitta, or *K* for Kapha in each circle according to the description best fitting each aspect.

To experience characteristics different from one's respective *doshe* might indicate a derangement of that *doshe*.

Reproduced with permission from *Ayurveda: The Science of Self Healing* by Dr. Vasant Lad, Lotus Press, a division of Lotus Brands, Inc., P.O. Box 325, Twin Lakes, WI 53181. ©1984 All Rights Reserved.

Now you have an idea what your doshic constitution is. Maybe you are mainly vata, maybe pitta. Or perhaps you are evenly vata and pitta with a minimum of kapha. No dosha is better or worse than another. An Ayurvedic doctor uses these categories to diagnose and treat disease, but in order to be more precise, the doctor also refers to fifteen subdoshas. For our purposes, we need only to focus on vata, pitta, and kapha.

Vata

As mentioned, qualities define doshas. The qualities of the vata dosha are:

- dry
- cool
- rough
- mobile
- erratic
- quick

Notice that, with the exception of "rough," these qualities could describe air. Therefore, think of vata as the "air" dosha. Anything that is predominantly characterized by one or more of these qualities is vata. The activity of breathing, which involves movement and air, is vata. Our nervous system, with its ultrafast nerve synapses, is vata.

On a psychological and spiritual level, vata enables us to express our emotions and be creative. People who are constitutionally vata tend to be very expressive and animated. They often have quick speech and talk with their hands. Overall, their movements are apt to be quick and erratic. Vata types learn quickly, but forget quickly, too. They have a tendency to be spacey. Those with a restless mind and an inclination toward insomnia are vata driven.

Certain physical characteristics are associated with each dosha, although most people have qualities from more than one dosha. People who are predominantly vata have fine bones and slender fingers and limbs. Generally, they are either tall or short and have a thin face. In addition, vata types are prone to have pale, dry, wrinkled skin that feels cool to the touch.

Doshas also apply to the times of day, seasons, and stages of life. During the day, vata is highest between 3:00 A.M. and 7:00 A.M. and also 3:00 P.M. and 7:00 P.M. When you wake before 7:00 A.M., vata energy propels you into action. The most vata season is from late fall to early winter. During this time, skin is inclined to dry out because an excess of vata permeates the environment. During our lifetimes, vata is highest from about age forty-five on. In earlier years, kapha and pitta dominate.

Once you get a feel for vata, you can identify the vata around you and in you. Stress is one of the great vata diseases of our day. Travel by planes, trains, and automobiles is vata because of the high-speed movement and the dehydrated air. An aerobic workout is a vata activity. A cold with a runny nose is vata. A soda cracker, which is light, airy, and dry, is a vata food, as is a raw carrot and that crunchy apple in the fruit drawer.

Too much or too little vata in the body provides a catalyst for change. I usually can tell when my vata is imbalanced, because my body, mind, and spirit exhibit certain symptoms. When I have a lot of errands to run and chores to do within a set amount of time, all of which require quick movements, my vata increases. Sometimes when this happens, I actually feel dizzy. If I sit under a cold draft in a restaurant, my vata increases and I get a runny nose. Watching television, particularly some of the channels geared toward kids, can be a very vata experience. The quick, flashing images rattle my nervous system.

Pitta

The qualities of the pitta dosha are:
- oily
- hot
- penetrating
- light (as in illumination)

Think of pitta as the "fire" dosha. Logically, it follows that pitta governs digestion; it is the digestive fire. As such, it also governs the absorption of food and regulates hunger and thirst. Pitta individuals are wont to have a healthy appetite and strong digestion. Furthermore, pitta regulates hormonal functions, which include metabolism and its biochemical and enzymatic processes, as well as body temperature.

Psychologically, pitta creates courage and joy, confidence and ambition, discrimination and understanding. With their penetrating minds and strong intellects, pitta individuals grasp concepts quickly, although they may not be good at remembering details like birthdays and anniversaries. They are passionate about their feelings and burn with their convictions, which they utter with clear and precise speech. Pitta people are natural leaders. Excess pitta can lead to irritability, anger, hate, and jealousy. Excess pitta may result in aggression and learning deficiencies. It also makes one overly competitive with a high need to win.

Pitta types are apt to have blond-to-reddish or copper-colored hair. Freckles and moles are often found on their skin, which is fair. If you are primarily pitta, you probably have good endurance and sweat profusely. Yet, as is typical of pittas, you may not tolerate heat well.

Pitta is highest from roughly 10:00 A.M. to 2:00 P.M. and then again from 10:00 P.M. to 2:00 A.M. Perhaps you have heard that it is best to have your biggest meal at noon. This is when the digestive fire reaches its peak. At night, you may feel brain dead by nine o'clock, but if you stay awake past ten, you begin to feel alert. That's because the universe's energy shifts to pitta around this time and stimulates mental capacity. The pitta season is summer, the season of highest heat, which provokes pitta. During one's lifetime, pitta is highest from puberty to about age forty-five, a time often devoted to higher education and career development, pursuits connected to pitta intellect. After age forty-five, vata becomes highest.

One of my daughters is very pitta. She craves winter, water, and cooler climates. If we drive around the desert in midday during the summer, she easily gets agitated. The heat unbalances her pitta, which is plentiful to begin with. When I'm expecting a visit from a pitta friend, I stock up on a treat like ice cream, which satisfies pitta with its sweet taste and cool quality. Although I, too, like cooling foods, especially in the summer, I've stopped drinking ice-cold water, lemonade, and iced tea with meals. In this country, unlike most others, our habit is to douse the digestive fires just before or during a meal. When we unbalance our digestive process, food may remain undigested in the intestines, becoming toxic.

Kapha

The last of the primary doshas is kapha, where qualities include:

- cold
- heavy
- slow
- stable
- dense
- hard
- smooth

Kapha is the "earth" dosha. It is the structure of the body—the bones, cartilage, and muscle. Like the earth, kapha is moist; it lubricates joints and tissues. The mucous membranes are kapha.

Kapha gives the body, mind, and spirit stability. It promotes calmness and makes us compassionate, caring, and content. Kapha people tend to be laid back; they are grounded and calm. Likewise, kapha is connected to security, a sense of identity, happiness, love, and satisfaction. It is very kapha to forgive. Kapha types may be slow to comprehend, but knowledge, once gained, is hard to nudge from their memories. Kapha people, with their tendency toward stability, do not readily welcome change in their lives.

Kapha types are built with bigger body proportions, like wide chests and large hands. Attractive, round, "bedrooom" eyes are very kapha. Kapha people have a tendency to carry extra weight. They have good stamina and are strong, even though they move slower and have slow digestion. A kapha appetite is not as large as a pitta appetite.

The kapha times of day extend from 7:00 A.M. to 11:00 A.M. and from 7:00 P.M. to 11:00 P.M. If you sleep in after a long night out and wake up at 10:00 A.M., you still may be tired all day. That's because you woke up during the kapha time of day when the energy is heavier. If you think of kapha as the earth dosha, it makes sense that spring, erupting with new, moist life, is the kapha season. Likewise, kapha is the predominant dosha in childhood, the springtime of our lives. Did you ever wonder why children move so slowly? They're in the kapha stage, which is characterized by slowness and heaviness. Children, in fact, are very connected to the earth, a kapha quality.

Like any dosha, kapha will increase if you participate in certain activities and ingest certain foods. Sit on the couch all day or take a vacation where you do little else but lounge in the sun, and your kapha will flourish. Actually, this type of vacation is very healing if you have a normally vata schedule—the kind where you are constantly on the go. The sun's warmth lowers vata and increases kapha. Heavy foods also raise kapha. The kapha in dairy products, for example, increases the kapha in the body, which in turn creates extra mucus. That's why it's best to avoid dairy foods during a kapha illness, such as a cold with a lot of phlegm.

Unbalanced doshas can result in disease. When an Ayurvedic doctor treats a patient, he first identifies the doshic constitution of the patient, and then determines the dosha of the disease. Chicken pox, for example, is a pitta disease. Some diseases, like arthritis or irritable bowel syndrome, can be vata or pitta or kapha, depending on the symptoms and the patient's constitution. The training and skill of the physician is critical in the treatment of such chronic diseases.

My Helen Keller moment of understanding the doshas occurred in Nepal when our group took a day off from lectures to journey into the Himalayan foothills. After a picnic lunch, our instructor held up a dried leaf that had fallen to the ground. He asked us what its primary dosha was. What do you think we said?

You have the rest of the chapter to mull it over. The answer is at the end.

BALANCING THE DOSHAS

Although our doshas naturally vacillate in and out of balance, an excess or depletion of any dosha can provoke disease. One way, therefore, to prevent disease is to keep the body's doshas relatively balanced. Proper nutrition is a very important way to do this on a daily basis. Usually we think of nutrition as the compounds found within food, but, in reality, its definition is much broader.

Ayurveda teaches how to nourish the body, mind, and spirit in diverse ways. Meditation, yoga, massage, and breathing techniques are healing to all doshas. Massage through the first seven years of life stimulates reflexes and tissue metabolism. A sesame oil massage is an excellent way to lower high vata. If your child bounces off the bedroom walls before bed, rub some sesame oil on the feet and a little on the navel. Try a sesame oil massage after a long plane or car ride. Traveling involves lengthy exposure to movement, which increases vata and unbalances the nervous system. Sesame oil reduces vata.

Ayurvedic physicians use herbal remedies extensively. Since I have discussed herbal medicine from a Western viewpoint, and since Ayurveda uses Indian herbs that most of us don't grow in our backyards, I am not going to explore this topic in detail. You may, however, find it beneficial to investigate this area on your own. Considerable research is being conducted on these herbs, which I suspect will soon become better known. You can order Ayurvedic herbs and herbal supplements from various companies.

Within the confines of your home, you will find it easiest to learn how to use food to promote your family's well-being. You can stock your refrigerator, pantry, and spice cabinet with the ingredients to help balance each dosha. Every infant, toddler, teenager, parent, and grandparent requires nutritious food for good health. Everyone can learn how to use this common denominator of nutrition to create and maintain balance on a physical, emotional, and spiritual level.

Nutrition and Food

Everything we eat affects the systems of our body. Consequently, appropriate food can be a powerful medicine. Food may not necessarily cure disease, but by balancing and enhancing the body's many functions it certainly can aid the healing process and even help prevent disease. If your child has a fever, for example, a diet that reduces pitta is beneficial. Fever, which is characterized by heat and inflammation, is a pitta illness. (Remember that pitta is the fire dosha.) In this circumstance, foods that lower pitta soothe and heal the body.

At the end of this chapter you will find a food chart reprinted from *The Ayurvedic Cookbook,* by Amadea Morningstar. This chart, variations of which are found in almost all books on Ayurveda, lists foods that increase and decrease each dosha. Take a minute to look up "apple." You will find it under "No ▲" in the vata column. Although somewhat juicy, apples are predominantly light, airy, and dry; thus, they aggravate vata. Notice that sweet apples decrease pitta, while sour ones increase pitta. All apples decrease kapha. They're a good pick-me-up snack when you feel heavy and lethargic but desire a sweet taste. That's when I gobble mine. If you feel chilled, a likely vata imbalance, you might take a few bites and toss it.

This chart is beyond my powers of memorization, so I keep the cookbook on the kitchen counter within easy reach. I don't consult it every day, but when the kids get a runny nose or I'm feeling too pitta or vata, I refer to it. I then can determine the kind of relationship that any of us will have with a particular food. In our family, we all are considerably vata. In the vata season of winter, for instance, a piping hot bowl of oatmeal with cinnamon and nutmeg is a balancing way to start the day. That's a healthy relationship.

If you try to use food to balance the individual doshas of each family member, you may go a little crazy. You may be more vata than your pitta husband or your kapha kids. You need a spreadsheet for that kind of planning. I find it much easier to cook a meal using foods that balance all the doshas. When someone has an acute illness, then I turn to foods that help bring a particular dosha back into balance.

Digestion

In Ayurveda, the pitta-driven digestive fire is called *agni*. If our agni cannot do its job correctly, half-digested food remains in the colon and becomes toxic. This toxic residue is called *ama*, which means "raw" and "undigested." According to Ayurveda, ama is a primary cause of many diseases. This doesn't mean that all disease can be traced back to the stomach or intestines, but rather that ama can create imbalance in the body's functions. The converse also holds true: an imbalance in the body's functions can create ama. The science of Ayurveda gives considerable attention to ways of reducing ama and ways of preventing ama buildup. As mentioned, proper diet is an excellent prevention.

Another reason to be aware of your digestion is that it is through digestion that our cells eventually receive what they need. Of course, they need vitamins, minerals, and other nutrients, but according to Ayurveda they also need the proper energy from food. In fact, all food contains energy, which is the life force present in everything. Ayurveda calls this energy *prana,* which is equivalent to the chi of Chinese medicine and the vital energy of homeopathy. So the body absorbs not only the chemicals in foods, but also food's inherent energy. If the colon is not functioning properly, it may not be able to absorb sufficient food energies. This concept is not recognized by Western dietetics. Food that is low in vital energy does not provide us with the necessary nutrition. Foods that are processed and full of pesticides or chemicals, or are left over for too long, lack this vital energy. The theory that food contains energies is found in Ayurvedic writings and the texts of classical medicines such as Traditional Chinese Medicine and Hippocratic Medicine. These writings say that food is most healing when fresh and whole. Hindus don't eat foods that are more than a day old because the energy in leftovers is thought to be minimal. Furthermore, fast foods are very low in anything vital. Such foods will not nourish our bodies in the same way as fresh, organic foods.

Some practitioners of Ayurveda, as well as other holistic philosophies, argue that microwaves seriously deplete food of vital energy. Because studies performed on microwaved food analyze chemicals and not vital energy, you won't find many references in scientific literature to the negative effects of microwaves. The only one that I was able to locate came from an article in the December 9, 1989, issue of the *Lancet.* According to the article, when milk samples were heated in a microwave oven, the amino acid L-proline was converted to D-proline, which is a known neurotoxin. The authors advised "further studies on the molecular changes of amino acids and other compounds because so little has been published about this aspect of microwave treatment."[1] Microwave ovens are now a standard kitchen appliance. Most likely, "further studies" on their detrimental effects has been minimal. Again, from a holistic standpoint, microwave ovens definitely are not in our best interest. When we finally decided to get rid of our microwave oven, four months after returning from Nepal, I went through a brief adjustment. I learned to heat baby bottles in a pan of water and to boil water in a teakettle. Now I'm only reminded of its absence when a visitor asks, "So where's your microwave?" I'm not inconvenienced in any way by not having one.

Spices

One way to assist digestion is to use spices. Ayurvedic food charts, like the one in *The Ayurvedic Cookbook* (see Table 6.2), indicate that many spices reduce kapha and increase vata. What these charts fail to reference, but the corresponding text addresses, is that spices promote digestion (agni). Here are a few spices and their effects:

Black Pepper
  • Balances all three doshas
  • Digestive stimulant, burns up ama
  • Kills parasites
  • Cleanses gastrointestinal tract

Cinnamon
  • Especially good for lowering vata
  • Warming

- Warms kidneys and therefore helps clear lungs
- Reduces muscle tension
- Strengthens heart

Coriander
- Cooling
- Especially lowers excess pitta
- Good digestive and absorbent
- Eases heartburn, dyspepsia, burning in stomach
- Good for diarrhea and dysentery

Garlic
- Tonic for vata
- Causes vata and pitta to move upward, so don't eat or take tablets of garlic with upper respiratory infections
- Good for digestive problems
- Works on all tissues; detoxifies
- Cleanses ama from blood and lymph systems

Ginger
- Increases agni
- When used with honey, decreases kapha; drink ginger tea with honey during illnesses that involve excess mucus
- Eases nausea and travel sickness
- Alleviates upper respiratory ailments

Turmeric
- Excellent for all doshas
- Increases digestion; particularly aids protein digestion
- Decreases ama
- Purifies blood
- Promotes proper metabolism
- Builds intestinal flora

Many foods sold in grocery stores, especially processed foods and even foods prepared in some restaurants, are spice deprived. Cooking with spices lends an element of creativity to the process. I enjoy experimenting with herbs and spices even though I don't always get the combinations or proportions correct. Like any skill, it takes practice. One place to start is with a cookbook that uses a myriad of spices in each recipe.

You can begin using spices when your child is an infant. When my youngest daughter was a baby, I added a pinch of cinnamon and nutmeg to her rice cereal. A small amount is sufficient; you don't want to bombard the baby's system with too much spice. When she started eating yogurt, I continued to add cinnamon. Yogurt is a very cooling food, so the warmth of cinnamon makes it easier to digest. Once, in a moment of laziness, I omitted the spice. After she finished eating the yogurt, Elle said in a distraught voice, "Mama, you forgot the cinnamon. I'm cold." I had never told her why I added cinnamon. I'm sure she noticed that the taste differed, yet she also noticed that the absence of cinnamon affected her physically.

In his book *Ayurvedic Healing,* Dr. David Frawley recommends warm, mild spices for children, including ginger, cinnamon, cardamom, coriander, fennel, turmeric, cumin, and basil. These all help regulate metabolism. To help clear mucus and strengthen mental and sensory functions, try basil, thyme, sage, hyssop, and mint.[2]

PURSUING AYURVEDA

Thus endeth this beginning lesson on Ayurveda. If you wish to expand your knowledge, check out some of the books in the recommended reading section. Should you decide to seek counsel with an Ayurvedic physician, you may be in for a little detective work or travel. In the United States, Ayurveda isn't practiced nearly as extensively as it is in India and Nepal. Nonetheless, if you or a loved one suffers from a chronic disease, it may be well worth the effort.

Oh, by the way, about that dead, dry, rough leaf we discussed earlier in this chapter: its primary dosha is vata. But you already knew that, didn't you?

TABLE 6.2

Food Guidelines for Basic Constitutional Types

Reprinted from *The Ayurvedic Cookbook* by Amadea Morningstar

▲ Aggravates Dosha ▼ Balances Dosha

	VATA		PITTA		KAPHA	
	No ▲	Yes ▼	No ▲	Yes ▼	No ▲	Yes ▼
FRUITS	Dried Fruits	Sweet Fruits	Apples (sour)	Sweet Fruits	Bananas	Apples
	Apples	Avocado	Bananas	Avocado	Grapefruit	Cherries
	Pears	Bananas	Grapefruit	Melons	Melons	Peaches
	Prunes	All Berries	Lemons	Oranges	Oranges	Pears
	Watermelon	Grapefruit	Strawberries	Pears	Watermelon	Raisins
		Grapes		Raisins		Watermelon
		Kiwi		Watermelon		
		Oranges				
		Strawberries				

NOTE: Guidelines provided in this table are general. Specific adjustments for individual requirements may need to be made, e.g. food allergies, strength of agni, season of the year, and degree of dosha predominance or aggravation. The guidelines are based on Dr. Vasant Lad's *Ayurveda: The Science of Self-Healing* (Lotus Press, 1984).

Fruits and fruit juices are best consumed by themselves for all doshas.

VEGETABLES	Frozen, Dried or Raw Vegetables Broccoli Cabbage Cauliflower Celery Eggplant Lettuce* Mushrooms Peas Potatoes (white) Spinach* Tomatoes	Cooked Vegetables Acorn Squash Carrots Cucumber Green Beans Onion (cooked) Potato (sweet) Pumpkin Zucchini	Beets Carrots** Eggplant Garlic Onions (raw) Onions (cooked)* Spinach ** Tomatoes Peas	Asparagus Bell Pepper Broccoli Fresh Corn Cucumber Celery Green Beans Lettuce Potatoes (sweet) Potatoes (white)	Acorn Squash Cucumbers Potatoes (sweet) Tomatoes Zucchini	Asparagus Bell Pepper Broccoli Fresh Corn Carrots Celery Green Beans Lettuce Onions Potatoes (white)
GRAINS	Cold, dry puffed cereal Corn Oat Bran Rye	Oats (cooked) All Rice Wheat Wild Rice	Corn Millet Rice (brown)**	Oats (cooked) Rice (basmati) Rice Cakes Wheat	Oats (cooked) Rice (brown) Rice (white) Wheat	Barley Corn Millet Granola Rice Cakes** Rye

* These foods are OK in moderation.
**These foods are OK occasionally.

TABLE 6.2 (CONTINUED)

	VATA		PITTA		KAPHA	
	No ▲	Yes ▼	No ▲	Yes ▼	No ▲	Yes ▼
ANIMAL FOODS	Lamb Pork Venison	Beef** Chicken or Turkey (white meat) Eggs Seafood	Beef Egg Yolk Lamb Pork Seafood	Chicken or Turkey (white meat) Egg White Shrimp*	Beef Seafood Shrimp Lamb Pork	Chicken or Turkey (dark meat) Eggs (not fried or scrambled with fat)
LEGUMES	Black Beans Kidney Beans Lima Beans Pinto Beans Soy Beans Soy Flour Soy Powder	In moderation: Aduki Beans Red Lentils Soy Cheese Tofu	Black Lentils Red Lentils	Black Beans Kidney Beans Lima Beans Pinto Beans Soy Products Tofu	Kidney Beans Soy Beans Cold Soy Milk Soy Cheese Cold Tofu	Black Beans Lima Beans Pinto Beans Red Lentils Hot Tofu*

SWEETNERS	White Sugar	Brown Rice Syrup Fructose Juice Concentrates Honey Maple Syrup Molasses	Honey Molasses	Brown Rice Syrup Maple Syrup White Sugar*	Brown Rice Syrup Fructose Maple Syrup Molasses White Sugar	Raw Honey Fruit Juice Concentrates (esp. apple and pear)
OILS		All oils are fine, especially Sesame	Almond Corn Safflower Sesame	In moderation: Olive Sunflower Sesame Walnut	Olive Safflower Sesame Soy Walnut	Almond Corn Sunflower (all in very small amounts)

* These foods are OK in moderation.
**These foods are OK occasionally.

TABLE 6.2 (CONTINUED)

	VATA		PITTA		KAPHA	
	No ▲	Yes ▼	No ▲	Yes ▼	No ▲	Yes ▼
DAIRY	Powdered Goat's Milk	All dairy OK in moderation	Salted Butter Buttermilk Hard Cheeses Feta Cheese Sour Cream Yogurt	Unsalted Butter Cottage Cheese Most mild soft cheeses Ghee Cow's Milk Ice Cream	Butter Cheeses of all kinds Cow's Milk Ice Cream Sour Cream Yogurt	Ghee Goat's Milk

CHAPTER 7

Eating Well in Spite of Our Food

Let food be your medicine and medicine be your food.

HIPPOCRATES

DIARY OF A FOOD-CONSCIOUS MOTHER

Monday, September 3

Oops. Life got a little hectic today. Neglected dinner plans until twenty minutes before two starving girls returned from gymnastics. Swore I had seen a jar of organic spaghetti sauce in the pantry. Must have been a mirage. At least they ate the grilled cheese sandwiches, steamed broccoli, and raw carrots and cukes.

Tuesday, November 3

Both kids' lunches came back from school almost untouched. How can they have the brain power to think in class? Are they scarfing up food from their friends? They beg for all this junky stuff with food coloring and I refuse to buy it. Mean old Mom. I bought ice cream today, though. Every family needs its occasional soul food.

Wednesday, December 3

Last day before Christmas break. Went to Elle's preschool party in the morning. Chamomile tea, apple juice, and cookies without refined sugar, all organic. The kids loved the spread. Went to Hannah's grade school for afternoon party. Soda, nachos, Cheetos, and sugary, frosted treats. The kids, hyper as could be, loved this spread, too. Felt like I had traveled between two planets but drove no more than 20 miles.

Thursday, May 3

Got myself organized. Made chicken stir fry before 5:00 softball practice so it would be ready for a late dinner at 6:30. A snack was handed out after practice. I was chatting and missed intercepting it. The red fruit punch and gummi worms dented the girls' appetites. Guess I'll eat stir fry for lunch tomorrow.

Friday, June 3

Went to the last-day-of-school pizza party. Decided to contribute 8-ounce water bottles. Hesitated buying them. Seemed like a dull treat for a party. Arrived after the kids had consumed pizza and sodas. They dove for the cooled water bottles. Wished I had bought more.

Saturday, July 3

Gotta regroup. The spinach enchiladas didn't go over well last night at dinner. Why didn't I feed these to the kids when they were toddlers? Elle wants to be a chef when she grows up, but she eats about five things. Maybe she'll write a book of 101 things you can do with yogurt. The sequels will cover broccoli, cucumbers, kiwi, and frozen waffles. Would an Eggo make a good frisbee?

Sunday, August 3

> *Struck it lucky with chicken and veggies in a tasty sauce. Perhaps the moon was in the perfect phase, the temperature optimal, and the seasonings just right. Who knows, but dinner was a hit. Only leftovers were clean plates. May our food miracles continue.*

FACETS OF FOOD

Each week consists of twenty-one meals and, depending on the number of children traipsing through your kitchen, about five hundred snacks. Eating nutritiously, creatively, and affordably takes considerable planning, all of which can be quite a challenge if you're busy with babies, chauffeuring kids, balancing an outside career, or dealing with finicky eaters. Yet food preparation is a fact of daily life. Sometimes donning an apron, uncorking the merlot, and cooking up a feast soothes the weary soul, while other times fetching a simple snack requires the strength of Popeye.

Regardless of our culinary moods, we want our children to develop a healthy relationship with food. These days, that can be a feat. According to a report in the *Wall Street Journal*, 1.7 million kids under age six eat at least one of their daily meals at a fast-food restaurant.[1] Grocers place at children's eye level sugary, low-fiber cereals that entice young consumers with a "surprise inside" or a picture of their favorite character. For every positive food fact that *Sesame Street* or *Blue's Clues* teaches, a commercial advertising artificially colored and processed foods pulls a child in a different direction. The average child watches between thirty and forty thousand commercials annually.[2]

How can we ensure that our kids eat right? If you're like me, you don't want to have to earn a Ph.D. in nutrition or biochemistry in order to figure out the best diet. While it helps to know some basics about vitamins, minerals, proteins, fats, and fiber when choosing foods, I have discovered that the principles of nutrition inherent in classical medicines such as Ayurveda, Traditional Chinese Medicine (TCM), and Hippocratic medicine offer practical and sound dietary guidelines.

Guideline #1:
Buy Whole Foods; Avoid Processed Foods

When I was in grade school in the late 1960s, the only sandwich I ever wanted in my lunchbox was liver sausage on white bread. The mushier and whiter the bread, the better. White bread contains white flour, which is made from the part of a wheat grain called the endosperm. Starch and protein are the predominant nutrition in the endosperm. The unused portion of the wheat grain includes the germ and the bran. The germ contains carbohydrates, unsaturated fats, protein, vitamins E and B complex, and other minerals, while the bran is rich in fiber. When wheat is processed into white flour, about twenty nutrients are extracted; "enriching" the white bread returns nutrients like iron, niacin, riboflavin, and folic acid, although less than half of the original nutrients are returned.[3] White flour is a classic example of a processed food, or partial food. Other common processed foods include milled white rice, fruit juices without pulp, refined oils, and refined white sugar.

Today, as my children peer into their lunch bags, whole foods are capturing the nutritional limelight. Whole foods include unrefined whole grains, fruits, vegetables, nuts, seeds, and beans. These foods contain less saturated fats and chemical food additives and are loaded with nutrients. Whole foods like garlic, celery, parsley, carrots, licorice root, soybeans, and flaxseed harbor beneficial nonnutritive compounds called phytochemicals, which are thought to be anticarcinogenic. Dark green and yellow vegetables teem with vitamins C and E and beta-carotene. These substances, called antioxidants, scavenge free radicals, the unstable molecules floating around the body that may play a negative role in cancer and chronic disease.

On the other hand, these components reveal only part of the story. Phytochemicals, proteins, and the other molecules in food interact to form a synergistic whole. All these pieces and particles coexist in precise patterns that are influenced by energy. (Western science argues that genes govern synergy; holistic traditions argue that energy governs genes.) An apple, a beet, and a carrot are unique, synergistic systems complete with living energy. As previously discussed, this energy is the chi of TCM, the vital energy of homeopathy, and the prana of Ayurveda.

According to holistic health systems, every food has its own energy fields and its own internal metabolic processes, both of which interact with the energy fields and the metabolic processes of other living organisms. In a world where everything is intertwined, this interaction is perfectly logical. By now, this concept may sound very holistic, and it is: every living organism, be it two-legged, four-legged, or no-legged, influences every other living organism. Hence, a food's subtle energy fields and metabolic processes nourish human energy fields and all the metabolic processes occurring in human tissues, systems, and organs. Foods that have stronger energy fields, like fresh, natural foods free of chemicals, nourish us more than foods with weaker energy fields like frozen, leftover, and processed foods.

One other concept of holistic nutrition is worth mentioning. The taste inherent in food correlates to the healing propensity of food. This idea is a real oddity in the field of Western nutrition. Yet taste has been used for thousands of years to heal disease. The concept of taste extends beyond the tongue and taste buds—different tastes contain different inherent energies. Ayurveda, for instance, defines six tastes: sweet, sour, salty, bitter, astringent, and pungent. The parallel in Chinese medicine is the five flavors: sour, bitter, sweet, pungent, and salty. The sour flavor, for example, enters the liver and gallbladder, while the bitter flavor enters the heart and small intestine. In other words, specific tastes can be used to treat specific diseases. Practitioners of Ayurveda and TCM learn to use the subtle energies of taste with great precision when treating disease. As the practices and beliefs of Eastern and Western nutrition blend, we should experience some amazing nutritional healing.

While energy concepts are not common to all theories of nutrition, almost all theories recommend whole foods. The first whole food to consider feeding your child is breast milk. Granted, not every mother is capable of breast-feeding or interested in doing so, but the benefits of breast milk are extensive. It is an easily digested whole food complete with immune-boosting nutrients and antibodies that infants have not yet developed. In one Canadian study, babies who were breast-fed contracted 50 percent fewer illnesses, including pneumonia, ear infections, blood infections, and meningitis.[4] Moreover, a baby who feeds at the breast of a relaxed mother— a mother comfortable with providing this form of sustenance— receives those unique, nurturing energies that penetrate body, mind, and spirit. Some women experience discouraging difficulties with breast-feeding, such as insufficient milk production, sore nipples, and breast inflammation (mastitis). Occasionally breast milk contributes to colic in an infant. Herbal medicine, homeopathy, TCM, and Ayurveda are modalities that can be very effective in correcting these imbalances. I wish I had known this as I endlessly rocked a colicky baby. Be sure to consult a practitioner of these modalities rather than devising treatments for yourself.

Guideline #2:
Avoid Unhealthful Food Additives

Having espoused the virtues of whole foods, I have to admit that consuming a diet of only whole foods is somewhat impractical. After all, foods like chicken breasts and tofu are partial foods; however, they have a high nutritional value and add variety to the diet. Rather than buy only whole foods, a more realistic nutritional guideline is to buy whole foods when possible and to avoid processed, unnatural foods. The only way to identify processed foods is to read labels. The presence of enriched flour, high fructose corn syrup, hydrogenated oil of any kind, and artificial flavorings and colors indicate a processed food.

With three thousand additives currently in use, completely avoiding them is almost impossible! Nevertheless, it is a goal worth working toward. Additives are either natural or synthetic. At first glance, natural additives don't seem to have many drawbacks. Albumin, for instance, a protein found in egg whites, is used as an emulsifier. Other natural additives purportedly enhance the nutritional value of food; vitamin D, for example, "fortifies" milk. Although such additives are nonsynthetic and safe, holistic nutrition contends that these substances behave differently when added to a food than when found within a synergistic whole. According to this line of thinking, the vitamin C in an orange differs from the vitamin C in a tablet or the vitamin C added to foods. Paul Pitchford points out in his book *Healing with Whole Foods: Oriental Traditions and Modern Nutrition* that "70 mg of vitamin C ingested in the form of parsley or broccoli (one cupful) may strengthen immunity more effectively than 700 mg of synthetic vitamin C."[5] Perhaps this concept sounds as difficult to digest as raw corn, but let it serve as another argument for pure, unadulterated whole foods.

In addition to natural additives, foods also contain synthetic additives. The FDA and nutritional experts sometimes disagree on the safety of these additives. Scientific studies, many of which are inconclusive, can't referee the debate. In some cases, synthetic additives were used for years and then banned after concrete evidence of their dangers surfaced. The FDA has eliminated fifteen food dyes and at least fourteen other additives from the market in this manner. The following list of potentially harmful additives includes only four food dyes, but some experts recommend avoiding all artificial food coloring, especially blues and greens. At this point, the long-term safety of many additives remains unknown.

- *Acesulfame-K, aspartame, saccharin, and sucralose.* Non-nutritive, synthetic sweeteners. (See Guideline #3 for a discussion of saccharin and aspartame.) Animal tests on acesulfame-K link the chemical to cancer. Found in chewing gums, instant coffee and tea, puddings, nondairy creamers. May be used more extensively in the future. Long-term safety of sucralose unknown.

- *BHA (butylated hydroxyanisole) and BHT (butylated hydroxytoluene).* Prevent oxidation and therefore retard rancidity in the oils and fats found in foods like cereals, chewing gum, bouillon cubes, potato chips, and cooking oils. Controversial chemicals because studies indicate they cause cancer. BHT is banned in England. Both easily replaced by safer additives such as vitamin E.

- *Monosodium glutamate (MSG).* Still used as a flavor enhancer, particularly in Oriental foods, even though people sensitive to it report headaches, chest tightness, burning sensations, wheezing, and nausea.

- *Propyl gallate.* Prevents oxidation. Often used in combination with BHA and BHT. Studies point to possible carcinogenic effects. Found in vegetable oil, meat products, chicken soup base, potato sticks, and chewing gum.

- *Sodium nitrite and sodium nitrate.* Preservatives found in bacon, hot dogs, bologna, smoked fish, corned beef, ham, and other processed and cured meats. Studies show they may cause cancer. Pregnant women should avoid.
- *Sulfites.* Prevent bacterial growth. Used in freshly cut and dehydrated potatoes, fresh shrimp, dried fruits, and wine. May cause breathing difficulties, especially in asthmatics. Banned in the United States from fresh fruits and vegetables.
- *Red No. 3.* FDA recommended this dye be banned, but political pressures prevented the ban. Possible cause of thyroid tumors in rats.
- *Red No. 40.* Most widely used food coloring. As with other dyes, may cause allergic reactions, cancer, or behavioral problems.
- *Yellow No. 5.* The only artificial food coloring required to be identified on food labels. Banned in Sweden and Norway but not in the United States. Found in gelatin desserts, candy, baked goods, soft drinks, ice cream, pet food, and other processed foods. May cause allergic reactions, particularly in aspirin-sensitive people.
- *Yellow No. 6.* Found in beverages, sausage, baked goods, candy, gelatin. May cause allergic reactions. Animal tests linked it to tumors of the adrenal gland and kidney.

In her book *Food and Healing,* Annemarie Colbin says that "there is perhaps no other single thing we do to food that affects its nutrient content and life-sustaining energy—and hence our health—as negatively as the addition of chemicals."[6] Because synthetic additives have a tendency to block a food's access to oxygen, life processes within the food grind to a halt. Like a life support system hooked up to a dying patient, preservatives artificially extend life. How natural is this? How much vital energy is in a food whose expiration date is a year from now? Are these foods healthy supports for body and mind?

Another growing concern pertains to the relationship between food additives and conditions like asthma, food allergies, eczema, hives, and attention deficit hyperactivity disorder (ADD and ADHD). In October 1999, the Center for Science in the Public Interest (CSPI) reviewed twenty-three of the best studies done since the mid-1970s on the relationship between behavior and diet. Seventeen of them revealed a strong link between behavioral problems (including hyperactivity) and food dyes, food additives, and, to a lesser degree, milk, wheat, corn, and the salicylates found in strawberries, tomatoes, and apricots.[7]

After its review, the CSPI issued a report requesting that the Department of Health and Human Services inform parents, school officials, and health care providers that diet may affect children's behavior. It also recommended that dietary changes should be considered as the first treatment in ADHD and other behavioral cases. The report encouraged more research into diet and behavior and suggested updating Web site information and literature, including a "pamphlet that the FDA co-sponsors with a food-industry association" that denies that diet affects behavior.[8]

Letters from a group of cancer experts and diet and behavior experts accompanied the CSPI's recommendations. The cancer experts cited a 1995 study done by the National Toxicology Program (NTP) that found that Ritalin, the stimulant drug most commonly prescribed to treat ADHD, caused benign and malignant liver tumors in mice. The NTP now calls Ritalin a "possible human carcinogen."[9] Since 1990 the production of Ritalin, 90 percent of which is consumed in the United States, has increased more than sevenfold.[10]

The side effects associated with Ritalin include reduced appetite, insomnia, stomachaches, weight loss, stunted growth, and Tourette's syndrome.

The tales told by parents of ADHD children sound nightmarish and many parents claim that Ritalin restores normalcy to a family disrupted by a child's deviant behavior. But perhaps before resorting to such a potent drug, diet therapy is worth a try. Dr. Doris Rapp, a pediatric allergist and clinical ecologist, has successfully used diet therapy with thousands of behaviorally disturbed children. In her book *Is This Your Child's World?* she advises that "a child who thinks unclearly or becomes uncontrollable because of sugar or food coloring should not eat a dyed sugary cereal for breakfast, drink a sweet red beverage just before an exam, or eat colored candy before playing sports."[11] Is this too simple a solution for some children's behavioral disorders? Maybe, but isn't it worth a try?

Guideline #3: Minimize Refined Sugar and Avoid Synthetic Sweeteners

In the 1994 movie version of *Little Women,* set during the Civil War, Winona Ryder's character, Jo, savors a special sweet treat: an orange. The family in William Faulkner's *As I Lay Dying,* set in the early 1900s, buys bananas as its sweet treat. These days, bananas and oranges do not qualify for most people as "special, sweet treats." We view them as nutritional fruits, full of potassium and vitamin C, respectively, that are available almost year-round in most grocery stores. Today's special sweet treats are the ones marketed in movie theaters, on television, and, as I recently noticed, on the handles of gas pumps. These treats, most of which are candy, come in bright, synthetic colors and are loaded with refined sugar, which is nothing more than calories devoid of vitamins, minerals, and vital energy.

The sweet taste is essential to life. According to Ayurveda, it stimulates the mind, builds tissues in the body, and creates deep satisfaction. We have, however, taken this holistic truth to an extreme. The average American consumes 147 pounds of sugar a year. One can of soda contains about 10 teaspoons of sugar. From 1983 to 1999, U.S. sugar consumption increased 28 percent, a gain associated with an increase in obesity—especially childhood obesity.[12] Parents and teachers claim that youngsters go bonkers when too much sugar enters their systems. Ironically, scientific studies don't always confirm this observation.

Sugar causes other problems, as well. In excess, it creates an acidic pH in the body, which encourages the growth of yeast. Furthermore, sugar leeches minerals, such as phosphorous, from the body. Phosphorous absorbs calcium; the less phosphorous, the less calcium entering tissues and systems of the body.[13] In addition, the sugar "low" following continual sugar "highs" may result in hypoglycemia. If this pattern repeats itself too often, diabetes may ensue.

If you pay close attention, you may be able to discern if your child is addicted or reacts negatively to sugar. I always knew that one of my daughters gravitated toward sweets and would eat them all day long if allowed. I started feeding her healthy sweets like bananas, carrots, beets, Jerusalem artichokes, squash, and sweet potatoes. She loves them. I also substituted natural sugars, like honey and maple syrup, for refined white sugar in recipes, although I don't always do this when baking. A number of nutritional books and cookbooks, including *Jane Brody's Good Food Book,* include charts illustrating sugar substitutions in recipes.

In addition to refined white sugar, synthetic sugar substitutes—including acesulfame-K, sucralose, saccharin, and aspartame—should also be avoided. (Saccharin and aspartame are marketed as Equal and Nutrasweet, respectively.) Despite approval by the FDA and the American Dietetic Association, synthetic sugar substitutes remain controversial. In animal studies, saccharin caused bladder and lung tumors.[14] The National Toxicology Program lists it as a likely carcinogen. Saccharin provides no energy to the human body, which is incapable of metabolizing it.

Aspartame, on the other hand, is metabolized, which is not necessarily a positive. It breaks down into 50 percent phenolalynine; 40 percent aspartic acid, which can cause brain damage in fetuses; and 10 percent methanol (wood alcohol). In the body, methanol is converted into formaldehyde—a neurotoxin—and diketopiperazine, a brain tumor agent. About 78 percent of all food complaints filed with the FDA involve adverse reactions to aspartame.[15] From a holistic standpoint, aspartame, like saccharin, is a nonorganic chemical devoid of any life energy. It has been associated with headaches and migraines, rashes, ringing ears, depression, insomnia, loss of motor control, seizures, anxiety, phobias, heart palpitations, nausea, diarrhea, abdominal pain, weight gain, excessive thirst, and increased infection, among other symptoms.[16]

Mary Nash Stoddard, who founded the Aspartame Consumer Safety Network, reveals alarming information about the sweetener in her book *Deadly Deception: Story of Aspartame*. For starters, the symptoms mentioned above do not correspond with any specific disease pattern, which makes it difficult to persuade the FDA to label aspartame as a harmful additive. Moreover, the cumulative effects of ingesting this chemical are not fully understood. If you drink a diet soda containing aspartame every day for one, five, or ten years, what does the aspartame do to your body? Few studies have included children, yet aspartame appears in hundreds of products geared to kids. Even children's over-the-counter and prescription medicines often contain this chemical. Augmentin, for example, is prescribed routinely for ear infections and strep. Available in 125-, 200-, and 250-milligram dosages, only the 200-milligram dosage contains aspartame at this time.[17] Try to steer clear of products containing aspartame. If your child has an occasional soda, as do mine, teach them to avoid the diet type.

A new synthetic sweetener called Neotame is waiting in the wings for market approval. Monsanto holds the patent for this chemical compound. According to Mary Nash Stoddard, Neotame is essentially aspartame but with dimethylbutyl added to make it seven thousand times sweeter than sugar. Dimethylbutyl is on the Environmental Protection Agency's list of most hazardous chemicals. Consumer beware: Stoddard calls the chemical an "extremely dangerous food additive/sweetener to be avoided at all costs."[18]

One has to wonder why we need chemical sweeteners that fall under the category of neurotoxin when plenty of natural sweeteners are available. It appears to be far safer to use molasses, pure maple syrup, honey, unrefined cane juice powder (Sucanat), fruit juice concentrate, rice syrup, raw cane sugar (turbinado sugar), and stevia.

Derived from a South American plant called *yerba dulce,* or "sweet leaf," stevia has garnered considerable attention in the past few years. Paraguay Indians used stevia leaves as far back as the sixteenth century for medicinal purposes and to sweeten foods. In the 1970s, Japan declared the calorie-free stevia to be a safe food additive. No adverse reactions have been reported in conjunction with its use. Because the United States had no domestic research on stevia, the FDA banned its use and importation from 1991 to 1995, after which it fell under the auspices of the Dietary Supplement Health and Education Act, which classifies all herbal plant products as supplements. Stevia is an herb, not a food additive.

Both the Hiroshima University School of Dentistry and Purdue University's Dental Science Research Group found that stevia suppresses the growth of plaque. Other studies show that it positively influences blood sugar levels, even in hypoglycemic and diabetic patients. Stevia may also counteract mental and physical fatigue, harmonize digestion, regulate blood pressure, and promote weight loss. In addition, the herb may be a good natural sweetener when the body has excess mucus, candida, or edema.[19] It is available as loose leaves, as well as in liquid and powdered form. At this time, it is not added to any commercially available foods.

Guideline #4:
Buy As Much Organic Food as Possible

One Internet article cautions, "Shop with the idea that the food store is a minefield."[20] Although disheartening, perhaps this admonition is not unreasonable, especially in light of what is done to our food. Strawberries, for instance, receive up to five hundred pounds of pesticides per acre. While a portion of sprayed pesticides can be washed from the outside of produce, chemicals inside produce can never be removed. The ramification of pesticides on children is cause for concern. In 1993 the National Academy of Sciences released a report titled *Pesticides in the Diets of Children and Infants*. Children, the report reminds us, have immature kidneys and developing immune, nervous, and brain systems that are much more vulnerable to the effects of pesticides than are adult organs and systems. Since most toxicity tests are conducted on adult males, the effects of pesticides on children are minimally documented.

Similarly, the long-term effects of growth hormones and antibiotics in nonorganic dairy and meat products remain unknown. Recombinant bovine growth hormone (rBGH), a genetically engineered hormone, is routinely given to most dairy cows in the United States in order to increase milk production. However, rBGH is banned in Ireland, Great Britain, the Netherlands, France, Belgium, Luxembourg, Spain, Portugal, Italy, Germany, Switzerland, Norway, Sweden, Finland, Denmark, Greece, New Zealand, Australia, Canada, and Israel.[21] The FDA approved rBGH before studies were done on the long-term, low-dose effects of this hormone. In humans, rBGH stimulates the production of a hormone called IGF-1, which has been shown to promote tumor growth as well as cause abnormal growth in infants and premature breast growth in children.

The use of antibiotics in dairy cows is just as frightening. The FDA has approved thirty antibiotics to be used on dairy cows. Antibiotic residue in milk could result in drug-resistant bacteria. Antibiotics are also administered to chickens, beef cattle, and pigs. In grocery stores, organic meats come from animals not treated with antibiotics. A package of chicken labeled "natural" or "pesticide free" is *not* organic. Boar's Head and Coleman meats are two brands that are free of hormones and antibiotics and in which animals are fed pesticide-free grains. When I started buying organic beef and chicken, my husband and I immediately noticed an improvement in taste.

Not everyone agrees that pesticides, hormones, and antibiotics in food are dangerous or even problematic. The Hudson Institute, a conservative research group, believes that organic crops do not yield enough produce to feed an overpopulated world and require too many acres of land. Plastics and pesticides are the way to a harmonious environment and an adequately fed world, claims Dennis Avery, author of *Saving the Planet with Pesticides and Plastic* and director of the Center for Global Food Issues, a branch of the Hudson Institute.

Supporters of sustainable agriculture believe differently. They contend that, given the opportunity, sustainable farming—with its emphasis on crop rotation, the cultivation of nutrient-rich soil, and use of nonchemical pesticides—could support a large population. Biodynamic farming is another agricultural alternative. Developed in the early 1900s by the Austrian Rudolf Steiner, a scientist, philosopher, educator, and founder of the holistic philosophy of anthroposophy, biodynamic farming views the farm as a whole, synergistic, self-contained organism. More recently, Masanobu Fukuoka, a plant pathologist, developed and successfully used natural farming on a large scale in Japan. This type of farming embraces four basic principles: no cultivation, no fertilizer, no weeding, and no pesticides. Fukuoka's book, *The Natural Way of Farming: The Theory of Green Philosophy*, details his holistic approach to agriculture. "Nature is entirely self-contained," he writes. "In its eternal cycles of change, never is there the slightest extravagance or waste." According to Fukuoka, human endeavors have "strayed far from the bosom of nature."[22]

The two aspects of organic foods that frustrate me are availability and cost. Organic foods chip away at the checkbook. Although we increased our family food budget, the prices still make me cringe. Furthermore, I have to drive farther to find them than I do conventional foods. When we lived in Wisconsin, one way we cut down on the organic grocery bill was by joining a sustainable farm co-op. Each week, we received fresh, organic farm produce for a reasonable price. The farm owners delivered the produce to a designated site that, in our case, happened to be a co-op member's home 2 miles away. The produce selection depended on that week's harvest. I learned how to cook vegetables that I had never been adventurous enough to buy, like celeriac, swiss chard, and kale. You can also save money by buying organic foods in local health food stores or co-ops or from catalogs that offer organic staples like flour, nuts, and popcorn (or whatever your family staples are). Recruit a friend, neighbor, or family member to split orders. Finally, check your local farmers' markets—many sell organic produce and other foods.

Just remember, organic food has a tendency to spoil faster than conventionally grown food because it doesn't contain preservatives that artificially extend the life of the food. That's actually a positive.

Guideline #5:
Minimize Genetically Engineered Foods

Making headlines left and right, at least at the time of this writing, are genetically engineered (GE) foods, also called genetically modified organisms (GMOs), Frankenfoods, biotech foods, or transgenic foods. In genetic engineering, genes from bacteria, viruses, and insects are inserted, or spliced, into plants. The new breeds of plants that contain these genes are resistant to certain pests or have different nutritional components. Advocates of genetic engineering maintain that it increases crop yields, prevents soil erosion, and, in some cases, lowers pesticide use. Furthermore, crops can be genetically engineered to resist the damages of herbicides still used to kill weeds. Multibillion-dollar chemical and agricultural companies, like Monsanto, have invested heavily in biotech research and eagerly promote the safety of GE foods, as does the FDA, various food industry organizations, and the American Dietetic Association (ADA).

Outcries against bioengineered crops reverberate around the globe. Too many harbingers of trouble have already surfaced, say the rivals of bioengineering. For example, bees that were fed proteins from genetically modified rapeseed had difficulty distinguishing the smells of different flowers.[23] Organic farmers have rallied against splicing genes from the *Bacillus thuringiensis* (Bt) bacterium into alfalfa, apple, broccoli, corn, cotton, cranberry, eggplant, grape, peanut, rapeseed, rice, tobacco, walnut, poplar, and spruce.[24] *Bacillus thuringiensis* is an effective natural pesticide frequently used in sustainable agriculture. A plant engineered with Bt genes continually produces large quantities of pesticide. The concern is that pests will develop resistance to Bt and spawn generations of superresistant pests. If this happens, the Bt sprayed on organic plants will no longer be strong enough to kill pests. Organic crops will suffer.

Since no long-term studies have been conducted, no one can say with absolute certainty that GMOs are not dangerous to your health, my health, or our planet's health. No studies have been conducted on infants who drink genetically engineered formula or children who eat GMOs. Thus far, no methods exist that measure the magnitude of risk for anyone consuming gene-altered foods. Are we humans the rats in the laboratory?

Question after question surrounds the issue of transgenic foods. Will history show that genetic engineering upsets ecosystems of plants and animals that have developed over millions of years? Is technology crossing natural boundaries that, in ways we may not yet fully understand, protect us, sustain us, and orchestrate our interconnected living? Does inserting a gene from one species into another affect the function of the new, modified organism? Can a foreign gene alter the substances in foods that now protect us against cancer? Can it cause new proteins to be formed that may harm us? Or cause allergies? As herbicide-tolerant genes appear in more and more crops and cross-pollinate with weeds, will weeds become herbicide resistant? Will greater quantities of herbicides then be sprayed on crops? Will biotech crops mate with wild neighbors and form uncontrollable crops? Will GE products increase antibiotic resistance? Will they encourage soil erosion and reduce soil fertility? Are we unwittingly sabotaging the very thing that keeps us alive—our food?

Various companies are responding to consumer demand for non–genetically engineered foods. Gerber and Frito-Lay, for example, now shun GE ingredients. In 1999 the British and Spanish divisions of Nestlé S.A. said that they would stop adding GE ingredients to products marketed in Britain and Spain, and the European Union issued a moratorium on genetically engineered crops. The largest soybean company in Japan, Fuji Oil Co. Ltd., no longer manufactures genetically engineered soy protein products, while the largest tortilla maker in Mexico refuses to import GE grain. Australia also has taken a stand against GE produce. In England, various consumer groups are recommending that people avoid all U.S. fruit, vegetables, ice cream, milk, milk powder, butter, soy sauce, chocolate, popcorn, chewing gum, health foods, and vitamins. Currently, unless a product carries a "certified organic" label you can't be certain if the product includes GE ingredients. A 1999 poll by *Time* magazine indicated that 81 percent of respondents want genetically engineered foods labeled.

Dr. John Fagan, a molecular biologist and former genetic engineer, vehemently criticizes the biotechnology that releases genetically engineered organisms into the environment or alters the human genome. In 1994 he returned a National Institutes of Health grant of $613,882 that was earmarked for genetic research. He also withdrew another grant application worth $1.25 million. In his words:

> We are living today in a very delicate time, one that is reminiscent of the birth of the nuclear era, when mankind stood at the threshold of a new technology. No one knew that nuclear power would bring us to the brink of annihilation or fill our planet with highly toxic radioactive waste. We were so excited by the power of a new discovery that we leapt ahead blindly, and without caution. Today the situation with genetic engineering is perhaps even more grave because this technology acts on the very blueprint of life itself.[25]

Guideline #6:
Minimize Irradiated Foods

Another technology designed with the intent of benefiting our food is irradiation. Foods are placed in an enclosed chamber and exposed to radiation, usually in the form of gamma rays emitted from radioactive cobalt-60 stored in stainless steel rods. Since the neutrons needed to make a substance radioactive are not emitted during the process, irradiated food does not become radioactive. The radiation—given at low, medium, or high doses depending on the foodstuff—kills certain pathogens in the food, including *E. coli,* listeria, and salmonella. Food viruses, however, are not killed, nor are some of the more virulent bacteria, such as the botulism bacteria. Besides being more sterile, radiated food sometimes has a longer shelf life than nonirradiated food.

In the United States, an estimated nine thousand people die annually from food-related illnesses, and another seven to twenty - thousand become ill. The ADA, the Centers for Disease Control and Prevention, and the World Health Organization support food irradiation as a means of reducing the incidence of disease caused by contaminated food. Furthermore, this technology may replace the practice of using highly toxic fumigants on conventionally grown food. About 170 irradiation facilities exist worldwide. American grocery stores are just beginning to offer irradiated foods—primarily poultry, fish, red meat, fruits, herbs, spices, and wheat.[26] Hospitals routinely serve irradiated food to seriously immunocompromised patients, such as individuals undergoing bone marrow treatments.

To anyone ever laid up with a bout of food poisoning, food irradiation may sound like a safe, preventive measure. However, opponents maintain that the process has too many potential problems and unanswered questions. Irradiated foods, particularly fruits and vegetables, may look prettier and last longer, but their flavor and texture sometimes change. Irradiation creates free radicals in the food, although the ADA claims that these "radilytic products" are no different than the free radicals that result from cooking, roasting, pasteurizing, and freezing foods. If you recall, free radicals are unstable molecules that may contribute to cancer and chronic disease. Irradiation also decreases the concentrations of B vitamins and ascorbic acid. Mice that were fed irradiated chicken had seven times fewer offspring than those fed cooked chicken. In fruit flies that were fed foods radiated at different doses, the incidence of death increased as the radiation dose increased.[27]

Will microorganisms mutate into strains resistant to radiation, as they have to antibiotics? Does irradiation kill the bacteria responsible for creating the foul smell that alerts us to spoiled meat and food? If we don't realize that our meat is spoiled and we eat it, are we in danger of more serious food poisoning from bacterial strains, like the botulism bacteria, that still inhabit the meat? Have sufficient long-term studies been conducted on humans? Does irradiated food affect human fertility? Most important, how is the energy—the chi—of the food affected? Are we consuming foods that have lost much of the vital energy needed to support us and keep us healthy? Perhaps we should concentrate on eliminating contamination during the early stages of food processing—including growing, raising, harvesting, storage, and manufacturing—rather than at the end stage.

If you want to avoid irradiated foods, look for the label that the FDA requires. Irradiated food packages must say "treated by radiation" or "treated by irradiation." They also are required to have a radura symbol: a flower inside a circle that has a solid line on the bottom half and is segmented on its top half. Unfortunately, restaurants, including those on cruise ships, in hotels, and in clubs, are not required to inform you if they are using irradiated foods.

Guideline #7:
Use Supplements Judiciously

Supplements are a megabucks industry that has spread from specialized health food and vitamin stores to doctors' offices, to Walgreens and Wal-Marts, and to every supermarket in between. Often, we view supplements as magic bullets able to cure illness or compensate for the sorry state of our food supply. Within conventional, alternative, and integrated medicines, however, debate rages about the need for supplements, the appropriate supplements to take, and their synergistic effects. Much remains unknown in this area. If we eat whole foods that are free of pesticides, antibiotics, and hormones, and we avoid partial, processed foods, do we need supplements?

Let's step again into the world of Chinese, Ayurvedic, homeopathic, Hippocratic, and anthroposophic medicines for a view of the body and mind. The first concept to remember is that the physical and emotional body is in constant flux. The body is inherently brilliant. Changes at any given moment are the most appropriate ones possible to establish *optimum balance.* Also recall that classical medicines speak in terms of patterns. Toxins, which are basically anything unnatural, disrupt healthy patterns. When disease patterns assert themselves, the weakened body may require outside assistance in order to reverse these patterns. The role of nutritional therapy is to assist the body and mind in transforming disease patterns back into healthy patterns.

What is adequate nutritional therapy? My husband has consulted a number of practitioners, who recommended a multitude of supplements. One even suggested taking fifteen supplements at one time. Gregg took about four supplements, but decided after a few months to stop because he felt more imbalanced than before. If you do take supplements, monitor how you feel. If the condition rectifies itself, take a break from the supplements: the body has righted itself and continued supplementation could again imbalance it. Anything taken in excess may have negative effects.

I've opted not to give my children, or myself, multiple vitamins or other supplements. I'd rather spend the money on organic, whole foods. During a specific illness, at the recommendation of our holistic doctor, we may use a supplement. Sometimes I use foods in cooking that are categorized as supplements. For instance, brewer's yeast (also called nutritional yeast) is a whole-food supplement rich in B vitamins, chromium, sixteen amino acids, and at least fourteen minerals. (We like its cheesy flavor on popcorn. Try it yourself: Buy organic popcorn and organic olive oil. Pour a few handfuls of popcorn kernels in a pan that has a lid. Then pour in enough oil to cover the kernels, place the lid on the pan, and cook over low heat. Sprinkle sea salt and brewer's yeast on the popped corn and you have a treat not to be beat!)

Guideline #8: Learn the Art of Food Preparation

This is where, if you are so inclined, you don the apron and crack the merlot. I have found considerable joy, as well as considerable frustration, in the art of cooking. There's no way around this one: we have to learn to cook. It's how fresh and healthy food gets prepared. Granted, I get lazy sometimes and buy a few organic frozen dinners or pizza, but I cook, too. I'm not an A1 chef, even though cooking is part of my daily routine. A few ideas have helped me so that I can at least prepare a number of tasty meals and enjoy most of the time spent in the kitchen.

- Use spices—lots of spices. Spices help digestion and add taste (energies) to food. Although the best cooking incorporates spices effectively, don't be afraid to make mistakes.
- In fact, make lots of mistakes in the kitchen. I've long stopped tallying my dinner flops. But every flop has taught me something.
- Find some mentors. I learn from my friends who are whiz-bang cooks. When I'm suffering kitchen burnout, I buy the food and invite them over to cook. New ideas, new inspiration.

- Find recipes that have ingredients you've never heard of, and then scout out those ingredients. That may mean going to a specialty store, like an Asian food market, or exploring the aisles of a health food store.
- Put together five or six meals that become no-brainers. When you're really pressed for time, you can whip these up quickly. I've learned to use a wok for a quick, easy way to cook meats and vegetables.

Guideline #9:
Eat with Reverence

The food is prepared, the table set, and the family gathered. Now comes the joy of eating. This is the spiritual side of food—the communing, the sharing, the discussion of the day's events. This relaxed gathering, with no TV blaring and no answering of phone calls, is part of our daily nutritional requirement. If we are what we eat, then best we keep our foods fresh, natural, and healthful and—just as important—learn to savor them.

CHAPTER 8

Environmental Concerns

The chemicals to which life is asked to make its adjustments are no
longer merely the calcium and silica and copper and all the rest of the
minerals washed out of the rocks and carried in rivers to the sea; they
are the synthetic creation of man's inventive mind, brewed in his
laboratories, and having no counterparts in nature.

RACHEL CARSON
SILENT SPRING

Sometimes the obvious takes a while to wedge into my awareness.
We had lived in our house for about a year when I attended a
seminar on indoor air pollution. One of the environmental experts
pointed out the drawbacks of having a garage attached to one's
house. That night, I parked the car in our garage-attached-to-the-
house and opened the door leading into the laundry room. Carbon
monoxide, carbon particles, nitrogen dioxide, and sulfur tagged
along beside me as I walked into the laundry room, then the kitchen
and the family room. I don't know why this pattern had never
caught my attention before—the strong fumes don't exactly qualify
as aromatherapy.

I've since noticed other things, too.

The day I was a mother helper at school coincided with building
maintenance day. I probably wouldn't have paid much attention to

the outdoor painting project had it not been for the white-suited moon men wearing protective hoods complete with clear plastic face coverings. Apparently, they were working with materials they didn't want to inhale or touch. As I escorted the second-grade class across the open commons, the workers, who were no more than 50 feet away, sprayed a liquid on walkway overhangs. We all got a good whiff of the chemicals. A chorus of "Yuck! It stinks!" and "What's that smell?" mingled with the noxious odor. By the time I reached the other side of the interior courtyard, my head ached. Later, one of the teachers said she could barely eat lunch in the teachers' lounge adjacent to the courtyard because the smell was so sickening.

Was it necessary to do this upkeep while school was in session? Did anyone consider how the materials being used would affect staff and students, particularly those with allergies, asthma, or chemical sensitivities?

Likewise, no one gave much thought to the way the indoor ice rink was being cleaned the day the kids and I went skating. An employee doused the Plexiglas surrounding the rink with a blue, ammonia-based window cleaner. The liquid dribbled onto the wooden railing that children and wobbly-ankled adults grabbed for support. The ammonia stung our nostrils, and anyone who touched the wet railing and later ate a snack probably ingested some of the cleaner. White vinegar, a proven disinfectant, and warm water would have done the trick without the toxicity. (Maybe public health codes should sanction vinegar as a disinfectant.)

Chemical Culprits and Challenges

We all know that chemicals permeate our world. Experts estimate that more than seventy thousand synthetic chemical compounds have settled into our water, air, and soil.[1] In light of our toxic mess, one might assume that we would proceed with extreme caution and use chemicals sparingly. Chemicals, however, have made us lazy. Insecticides, herbicides, and fungicides quickly eliminate pests from yards and gardens. Industrial chemicals such as dioxin, PCBs, mercury, lead, cadmium, alkyl phenols, pthalates, styrenes, formaldehyde, benzene, ammonia, and chlorine have countless applications, ranging from carpet installation to the bonding of building materials to the cleaning of homes, businesses, and schools. Without a doubt, chemicals are big business.

Yet only 2 to 10 percent of commercial chemicals have been tested for safety on adult humans.[2] Rarely is testing done on children, whose developing bodies tend to be far more sensitive to foreign substances than adult bodies. Many chemicals stimulate or block estrogen and other hormones. These endocrine disrupters may be related to an increased incidence of early puberty in children and infertility, lower sperm counts, testicular cancer, and breast cancer in adults. Furthermore, scientific studies have yet to verify how our excess of chemicals affects our central nervous systems, immune systems, and limbic systems and how our bodies integrate or eliminate chemicals. Also unanswered is the mystery of how chemicals interact with each other.

When under sufficient pressure from scientists and citizens, the government may ban a chemical from the marketplace. But the culprit may linger in our surroundings for decades. This is what happened with the pesticide DDT. In 1939 Swiss chemist Paul Müller discovered that DDT poisons the nervous system of insects; therefore, it could be used as an insecticide. During World War II, the military sprayed DDT over bug-infested areas just prior to invading them. Following the war, the chemical was used extensively to reduce insect-related diseases, like malaria and yellow fever. In the United States and elsewhere, farmers used it to double crop production. The detriments of DDT caught the public's eye in the 1960s.

Rachel Carson's 1962 exposé *Silent Spring* brought to attention insects' growing resistance to the chemical. She also publicized the theory that DDT was permeating the food chain and disrupting reproduction, even in humans. The government finally banned DDT as an active ingredient in 1973. Traces of it still appear in soil, water, homes, and even breast milk.

All this talk of toxic chemicals can spark more than a few flames of fear, not to mention anger. You may wonder if you should run out this instant to purchase a gas mask. I'm not dishing out these statistics as a scare tactic, however. The facts are frightening, because they illustrate the seriousness of our predicament, but their primary purpose is to create awareness, without which nothing will change. Once we are aware that change is needed, we have a choice: institute change or maintain the status quo. Solving the problem of air, water, and land pollution requires a team effort of citizens, environmentally concerned organizations, businesses, and elected officials. Without a doubt, we need to join such teams. We can also work individually at minimizing toxins in one area central to our lives. That area is the great indoors.

According to the EPA, we spend 90 percent of our time inside.[3] Likewise, our children spend the majority of their time within the walls of home, day care, or school. Unfortunately, indoor air has become alarmingly polluted, particularly from chemicals—both synthetic and natural. Studies indicate that children and adults who live in homes with poor indoor air quality experience increased allergies, coughing, wheezing, shortness of breath, asthma, bronchitis, upper respiratory tract symptoms, headaches, eye irritation, muscle aches, fever, chills, nausea, vomiting, and loss of concentration.[4] Since the federal government is only beginning to set standards for indoor air quality in private residences, schools, and even public places such as movie theaters, libraries, malls, office buildings, and buses, the responsibility of tackling this problem is ours. By making a few simple modifications within our living, work, and school environments, we can decrease the potential for future health problems.

CHEMICAL CULPRITS

You probably know that in homes and other buildings, lead, asbestos, and radon have been assaulting human health for years. For example, radon, a natural gas strongly linked to lung cancer, is thought to be present in over six million homes at unsafe levels.[5] (You now can hire professionals who will test for radon in your home or you can purchase long- or short-term testing kits at hardware stores or via mail order.) In addition to these well-known chemicals, volatile organic compounds (VOCs) are attracting attention. Dr. Doris Rapp, who specializes in allergies and environmental medicine, forecasts that VOCs "will become a household word within the next few years because they are so prevalent and damaging—and at times, even deadly."[6]

A VOC is a compound containing carbon. The reason that these organic compounds, also called organic chemicals, are called "volatile" is because they remain active in the products that contain them. They escape into the air, both when the product is used and when it is stored. Volatile organic compounds include acetone, found in nail polish remover; pthalates, found in plastics; benzene, found in adhesives and air fresheners; formaldehyde, found in particle board and pesticides; and hundreds of other compounds. So many VOCs abound that this book would require pages and pages of fine print to list them all.

Volatile organic compounds are some of the worst toxins that we can encounter, and they surround us both indoors and outdoors.

When the compounds escape from the products that contain them—such as furniture polish, glue, and air fresheners—they adhere to dust and other airborne particles. These particles then settle on our clothes, furniture, carpets, and even our skin. The EPA has determined that the levels of at least a dozen common VOCs are two to five times higher in the home than outside, regardless of whether the home is located in a rural or urban area.[7]

A quick cruise through the bathroom reveals the prevalence of VOCs. The disinfectants under the sink and the air freshener on the toilet emit VOCs. Those cosmetics in the drawer very likely release formaldehyde, benzene, toluene, and methyl and ethyl compounds. When used, the perfume and cologne on the counter outgas, or emit, VOCs. Many fragrances, such as those found in facial tissue, deodorant, shampoo, soap, and sunscreen, all release VOCs. In addition, the carpeting covering the floor, the paint on the wall, and the varnish on the wood trim expel VOCs. Even that new vinyl shower curtain constantly releases VOCs. In fact, you can probably smell the organic compounds. As you might have guessed by now, we touch and breathe VOCs all day long. We even ingest them: mouthwash, coffee, eggs, and many food additives contain formaldehyde, one of the most prevalent VOCs in our environment.

Currently, the federal government does not require manufacturers to label the VOCs used in their products. This information is classified as confidential business information and, as such, is exempt from disclosure. On some packages, VOCs are listed as "inert ingredients." Do not confuse the dictionary definition of "inert"—"lacking the power to move"—with the word as it appears on labels. Inert ingredients serve as solvents for a product's active ingredients. These active ingredients are dissolved in the inert ingredients. Although the inert ingredients often are VOCs that outgas into the air, the law does not require that labels list them.

"Yeah, yeah," the skeptics utter. "These chemicals are everywhere. But you don't exactly hear about people dying from exposure to them. The human race is still alive and taking showers without being asphyxiated."

Of course, one vinyl shower curtain isn't going to put anyone six feet under. The cumulative load of low doses of chemicals is the main concern. Do health complications result from long-term exposure to these low doses of chemicals? Right now, nobody has the answer to that question. Although the government has established the toxic exposure levels for certain chemicals, the consequences of constant exposure to low doses of VOCs and other chemicals have not yet been ascertained. Nevertheless, an increasing number of scientists, medical professionals, and consumers believe that repeated exposure to low doses of chemicals negatively impacts our health. Over days, months, and years, our bodies are forced to deal with thousands of VOCs, as well as inorganic compounds such as heavy metals, and gases such as carbon monoxide. Many of these compounds are thought to be toxic to the immune system. Hence, reducing the load of chemicals on the body can only be a preventative health measure.

SOLUTIONS

Fortunately, you can take measures to lessen your exposure to chemicals, particularly in your home. More and more retailers now sell "eco-products" that contain minimal or no VOCs and other chemicals. Organic shampoos, nonchemical cleaners, special filters for ducts, furnaces, and air conditioners, and even mattresses made with organic cotton are among the growing array of environmentally sound products. Look for retailers in your area who carry these products. Some stores specialize in products specifically designed for people with allergies, asthma, and chemical sensitivities. You can also order many products through catalogs. Check the Resource section at the back of this book for ideas of where to find eco-retailers. These options may be worth exploring, particularly if anyone in your household has a weakened immune system or respiratory disorders like allergies and asthma.

Purify the Air as Much as Possible

The most inexpensive way to remove VOCs is to ventilate your living space with fresh air. Open your doors and windows as often as possible. The circulating outdoor air helps remove many indoor pollutants. In addition, stop using products that increase indoor air pollution, such as aerosol cans. If you use products that contain toxic chemicals or VOCs, like varnish, make sure you use the products in a well-ventilated area.

Try to avoid perfumed products, a difficult task, indeed. Magazines, bills, car washes, cosmetics, foods, and even magic markers and crayons assault us with scents. Over four thousand different ingredients, many of them synthetic and about one-third suspected to be toxic, are used in fragrances. For example, acetone, ethanol, and methylene chloride are chemicals frequently found in cologne, perfume, and shampoo. The EPA classifies all three chemicals as hazardous waste. Unfortunately, the fragrance industry remains unregulated. New scents enter the marketplace at an alarming rate, but most are never tested for safety. A perfume-free product will carry the label "Free from all perfumes." However, a product with a label that reads "Perfume free" may not actually be perfume free; it may contain small amounts of fragrances or masking agents.

If at all possible, avoid dry cleaning. Most dry cleaners use perchloroethylene (PERC), which is a toxic solvent, hazardous air pollutant, and probable human carcinogen. The skin readily absorbs PERC from clothing. Environmental experts recommend airing out dry-cleaned clothes, although this will not remove all the PERC. You may want to try professional wet cleaning, now provided by more than 150 cleaners. Greenpeace's Web site lists these businesses.[8]

One item to consider purchasing is an air purifier, a machine that cleans air by removing particles and gases. Most people who purchase purifiers feel that they help reduce respiratory infections, asthma symptoms, and allergies. An air purifier should contain three filters: a pre-filter, a HEPA filter, and a carbon filter. The latter needs to be in the middle in order to collect gases. Because not all air purifiers are designed to collect gases, make certain that the one you purchase has this capability. When choosing a purifier, remember to include filter replacements in your budget. Generally, filters need to be replaced two or three times a year.

A vacuum cleaner with a HEPA filter removes as much as 99.97 percent of particles from carpeting. Regularly vacuum your soft furnishings, such as sofas and chairs covered in fabric, because dust and other particles settle on them.

Last, buy indoor houseplants. Green plants purify the air. NASA determined that the following plants significantly remove formaldehyde, carbon monoxide, dust, benzene, and trichloroethylene:

- Chinese evergreen (*Aglaonema* 'Silver Queen')
- Spider plant (*Chlorophytum elatum*)
- Pot mum (*Chrysanthemum x morifolium*)
- Janet Craig dracaena (*Dracaena deremensis* 'Janet Craig')
- Striped dracaena (*Dracaena deremensis* 'Warneckeii')
- Corn plant (*Dracaena fragrans* 'Massangeana')
- Red-edged dracaena (*Dracaena marginata*)

- Elephant's ear philodendron (*Philodendron domesticum oxycardium*)
- Heart-leaf philodendron (*Philodendron scandens oxycardium*)
- English ivy (*Hedera helix*)
- Banana tree (*Musa*)
- Reed palm (*Chamaedorea seifrizii*)
- Gerbera daisy (*Gebera jamesonii*)
- Golden pothos (*Epipremnum aureum*)
- Snake plant (*Sanseveiria trifasciata 'Laurentii'*)
- Peace lily (*Spathiphyllum 'Mauna Loa'*)[9]

Reduce Formaldehyde Exposure

As mentioned, one notorious VOC is formaldehyde, a suspected human carcinogen and possible toxin to the central nervous system. According to the National Academy of Sciences, 10 to 20 percent of the general population may react to extremely low concentrations of this chemical.[10] When emitted from products, formaldehyde can cause nasal stuffiness, itchiness, watery eyes, headaches, tiredness, insomnia, dizziness, and rashes, among a host of other symptoms. Formaldehyde is found in adhesives, air fresheners, car exhaust, carpets, chewing gum, coffee, deodorants, eggs, permanent press fabrics, insulation, mascara, shampoo, varnishes, vaccine preparations, wallpaper, and hundreds of other products.

Although you cannot avoid formaldehyde, you can decrease its potential to irritate. Products release more formaldehyde when they are new, when a building is tightly sealed, and when the air is humid. A baking soda wash will remove formaldehyde odors from furniture and cabinets made with particleboard. Simply mix ½ cup baking soda in 1 gallon warm water and wipe down the area with a sponge. This method can also be used on vinyl products like tablecloths and shower curtains.

Arts and Crafts

One of my daughters received red potter's clay for a birthday present. It was purchased at a specialty toy store and came packaged in shiny, thick foil. As soon as she opened the package, we could smell the clay. The scent was not fragrant, nor did it have an earthy smell like the clay used by professional potters. Because the ingredients were not listed, I had no idea what the odorous material contained. Whatever it was, it irritated noses and stained hands orange.

Arts-and-crafts materials often contain VOCs and other chemicals. The Labeling of Hazardous Art Materials Act of 1988 helped identify many children's art materials, such as crayons, chalk, paints, and modeling clay, that contain toxic substances. If the ingredients are not listed, look for the phrase "Conforms to ASTM D-4236," indicating that the material does not emit enough toxic chemicals to be an immediate hazard. The legislation, however, does not force manufacturers to eliminate all toxins from art and hobby supplies—many of which carry low doses of VOCs—nor does it require that labels indicate the presence of VOCs. Permanent markers, for instance, do not carry toxicity warnings. But have you ever smelled one? Whew! That odor comes from the emission of VOCs such as xylene, another suspected carcinogen. If you need to use markers, glues, other bonding materials, paints (even the oil paints included in paint-by-number kits), decoupage, or coatings of any kind, try to do so outdoors or in a very well ventilated area.

You can inexpensively make your own art materials. Children are usually very eager to measure and mix the ingredients for playdough, clay, and paints. Look for recipes in books like Annie Berthold-Bond's *Better Basics for the Home: Simple Solutions for Less Toxic Living.* Also, parenting magazines print ideas for making simple and safe art materials.

Use "Green" Household Cleaners

Pick up five or six cleaners in the grocery store and read the ingredients. "Hey, what ingredients?" you ask. You're right, most of them are not listed. But you do see "CAUTION," "HAZARDOUS," or "KEEP AWAY FROM CHILDREN," statements that are required by law on products that children can ingest. Most likely, these products contain VOCs. Cleaning supplies are a prime source of volatile organic compounds. Regardless of whether anyone in your home suffers from asthma or allergies, maintaining a toxin-free home is healthful. By changing to natural cleaners, you don't have to worry about children ingesting chemicals or inappropriately mixing cleaners that create toxic gases. A number of companies, like Ecover and Harmony, the latter of which markets products under the brand name Seventh Generation, sell nonchemical cleaning products. I also discovered that I can mix my own cleaning solutions at home and save money in the process.

If you've never made your own cleaners but are interested in giving it a go, start simple and experiment. Here's a few ideas to get you started on those weekly chores of dusting, vacuuming, laundering, and scrubbing. (Well, at least in theory they should be done weekly. Remember that VOCs not only remain free in the air, but also attach to dust particles, which then settle on furniture, floors, draperies, and knickknacks. Regular dusting and slow vacuuming helps remove them.)

The basic cleaning supplies to keep on hand include:

- Borax
- Baking soda
- Bon Ami (a natural scouring powder)
- Lemons

- Olive or linseed oil
- White distilled vinegar

These products should be available at most supermarkets. If you're not sensitized to smells, you also may want to buy a few essential oils. Oil of thyme and tea tree oil have antibacterial properties. Lavender oil and lemon oil smell fresh and yummy. Add a few drops of the oil to your cleaning solutions.

So you've got the goods. Now put them to use.

- *Furniture polish:* Mix 2 tablespoons fresh lemon juice with 2 tablespoons high-quality olive oil (linseed oil also works). Because lemon juice turns rancid, discard any unused mixture. I couldn't believe how well this one worked the first time I used it.
- *Window cleaner:* Add ½ cup vinegar to 2 cups water and store in a spray bottle. Wiping with newspaper or a squeegee will streak less than with a cloth. Do not add an essential oil because it will streak the glass.
- *Wood, tile, and linoleum floors:* Mix 1 part vinegar to 4 parts water. If linoleum is heavily soiled, pour 2 cups club soda in a spray bottle. Spray floor, and mop clean. Or sprinkle Bon Ami on a wet sponge and gently scrub soiled area.
- *Toilet bowl cleaner:* Add equal parts vinegar and baking soda—about ½ cup of each—to toilet bowl. The vinegar activates the carbonates in the baking soda and creates a pleasant-sounding fizz. Add essential oil and let sit in bowl for 15 minutes. This concoction also removes blockages from drains.
- *General bathroom cleaner:* Sprinkle Bon Ami on area to be cleaned and wipe off with wet sponge or cloth. Works well on kitchen sinks, too. On plastics, fiberglass, and imitation

marble, sprinkle Bon Ami on sponge first, add water, and
then wipe surface.

- *Laundry:* Use 1 cup borax per large load. For heavily soiled
  loads, use a detergent, but only half as much as you normally
  do. Add ½ cup baking soda.

You can expand on these suggestions by referring to the many
available books brimming with ideas for natural home care and personal care products.

Pesticides

Here in Arizona, people routinely spray their homes and yards to
keep out creepy-crawlies like millipedes, spiders, and crickets, the
latter of which are prime meals for scorpions. When I found a black
widow's nest in our garage near the kids' bikes and another one near
the front door, I decided to call a friend who has a Ph.D. in ento-
mology and owns a pest-control company specializing in integrated
pest management (IPM).

When Gordy came to the house, he first checked its perimeter for
spaces where pests could enter. Did the garage door sit tightly
against the driveway or could insects crawl in and then find a way
into the house? Were vents sealed properly? Indoors, he set baits—
little tents of paper with an adhesive on the bottom. These bait sta-
tions monitored the flow of insects in a particular corner, room, or
cabinet. He said that he would check the baits each week for a
month or two. He did not use pesticides inside. Most problems
could be solved with natural ingredients. Boric acid mixed with
peanut butter grease, for example, affects the physiology of ants and
eventually kills them.

When done correctly, IPM is a bit more labor intensive than
merely spraying pesticides indoors and outdoors. With IPM, chemicals are a last resort. Gordy sprayed a low-toxicity pesticide on the

three black widow's nests on the outside of the house. He did not spray in the garage, because the children's toys were there. (By then, we had destroyed the black widow's nest.) He never sprays indoors. Pesticides, even used in an enclosed area like under the kitchen sink, dissipate into the air and land on dust particles, which in turn settle on the toys that babies chew on and the floors on which babies crawl. Studies have found that children living in homes where pesticides were regularly used were six times more susceptible to cancer.[11]

Gordy only sprayed the perimeter of our house once, and that was three years ago. Sure, we've seen occasional crickets and spiders and a few millipedes since then, but no insects have come in droves. If they do, I will certainly call him back.

Environmental Illness

When my friend Barry moved into his condominium, he was a healthy thirty-nine-year-old. During the next twelve months, his health degenerated. First, he lost his sense of smell. Then an avalanche of symptoms descended on him, including migraines, digestive disorders, insomnia, weight loss, depression, and fatigue so severe that he finally quit working. Barry spent over ten thousand dollars trying to identify his illness. A battery of diagnostic tests failed to detect the problem. He even thought to have the air in his condominium tested for impurities. It registered safe and sound. Finally, Barry's exasperated internist and allergist sent him to a psychiatrist, who pronounced him thoroughly competent, but thoroughly angry.

Twelve months into the ordeal, Barry went on vacation and felt noticeably better. That's when the light went on: something in his condo was making him ill. He decided to pack his bags. While cleaning out the items under the sink in the master bathroom, he just about passed out. There, in a darkened corner, sat an uncovered canister of blue toilet bowl crystals containing chlorine. For an entire year, Barry had breathed in low levels of chlorine vapors for seven or eight hours a night. As a result, he developed multiple chemical sensitivity (MCS), a type of environmental illness where chemicals, even in low doses, trigger a myriad of symptoms.

The growing number of children and adults who suffer from an environmental illness underscores the dangers of chemicals. Some victims, like Barry, develop MCS after exposure to low levels of chemicals. Others link the onset of their illness to a specific toxic exposure. Roger, for instance, became dizzy and nauseous after spending five minutes in the back of a truck containing grapes sprayed with sulfur dioxide. Within months he was so chemically sensitized that the chlorine in his shower water made him vomit.

The proliferation of environmental illnesses such as MCS has given rise to a controversial "medical subculture" called clinical ecology.[12] Within the wards of mainstream medicine, this specialty barely receives a courteous nod. Organizations like the American College of Occupational and Environmental Medicine, the American College of Physicians, and Centers for Disease Control and Prevention refuse to classify MCS as a disease. Part of this reluctance stems from a scarcity of facts. Scientific studies have not adequately explained the body's physical mechanism that triggers MCS. Furthermore, chemically sensitive patients are difficult to treat because their symptoms involve more than one organ system. Symptoms may include respiratory problems, joint and muscle pain, gastrointestinal problems, skin disorders, insomnia, memory impairments, loss of concentration, depression, and fatigue, many of which do not respond to conventional treatments and require the care of more than one specialist. Because anxiety, depression, hyperactivity (particularly in children), and other psychological disorders are common with MCS, patients are often told to seek psychiatric help. "It's all in your head" is a common refrain.

While debate rages over the status of MCS, clinical ecologists and MCS patients must contend with reality. Pam is the mother of two daughters who both have MCS. Homeschooling is a must, since neither child can tolerate the chemicals in schools. Even a simple outing to a public park is infeasible because the girls react so strongly to pesticides sprayed on the grass. Meeting friends has become virtually impossible. These children lead very secluded lives. Sadly, this social isolation commonly challenges MCS patients. At this time, the best treatment for MCS is to avoid the problem—the chemicals that trigger symptoms. Many MCS sufferers are forced to build homes of nontoxic materials and eat only organic food. Clothing made with organic cotton may be the only fabric that does not provoke symptoms. In some cases, these expensive alternatives leave individuals and families destitute. They lose their life savings, life possessions, and—most upsetting—their lifestyles.

What You Can Do

Dr. Doris Rapp, a pediatric allergist and clinical ecologist, treats hundreds of children plagued by environmental illness. She well knows how tricky diagnosis can be. In her eye-opening book *Is This Your Child's World?*, Rapp offers steps that anyone can take to detect a potential environmental illness. She writes: "The downhill course in the learning ability of some environmentally ill children and the careers of many capable adults can be totally reversed by the actions of one caring, knowledgeable individual. Maybe that person can be you."[13]

First, observe your child after he touches, breathes, or eats something. Does your child feel differently, behave differently, or seem to think differently? For example, compare how your child behaves before entering his bedroom, day care, or classroom. Does his behavior change while he's in that space? How about after leaving the room? Does he get a headache or a stuffy nose after touching a certain type of fabric? Does he become hyper after eating strawberries or a snack with synthetic food coloring in it? You may want to record your observations in a notebook.

Certain symptoms may herald an allergy. Does your child ever have red earlobes, black eye circles, puffiness below the eyes, or red cheeks? Does she ever rub her nose, wiggle her legs uncontrollably, clear her throat repeatedly, or make clucking sounds in her throat? Are these symptoms present when your child is at home, or school? When do they disappear or reappear? Again, make sure to record your observations.

In addition, check your child's handwriting and/or drawing. Dr. Rapp suggests having your child draw or write before each class, snack, or chemical exposure. If you suspect an allergy to a certain substance, have your child write or draw upon exposure to that substance. Allergic reactions can alter handwriting.

Bear in mind that reactions to chemicals (and foods) can vary. Some symptoms occur within minutes of an exposure; others occur within an hour, or even longer. Likewise, symptoms can last for a few minutes or hours or even days or weeks. Your carefully recorded observations may reveal a pattern that points to the chemical or food causing the physical or emotional problems.

OUR ENVIRONMENTAL LEGACY

Fifty years ago, did anyone foresee that at the turn of the twenty-first century, thousands of toxic chemicals would permeate our air, water, and soil? Not even our living spaces are free from pollutants. Many illnesses, from asthma to allergies to MCS, are suspected of being provoked or caused by environmental factors. Ironically, as more children and adults fall prey to environmental illnesses, an increasing amount of chemicals continue to be manufactured, sold, and used.

Is this the legacy we will leave for our children? For now, I suppose, it is. I learned long ago, however, never to quit running until you're ten feet beyond the finish line. It is not inevitable that we will bequeath our children or grandchildren a toxic world. We certainly have the ability to clean up after ourselves. Are we motivated to do so? Rather than using our inventive minds to develop more synthetic chemicals, let's use them to create a healthy world. Even switching window cleaners from an ammonia-based solution to vinegar and water is a change for the positive. Little changes do count. So do little people. Let's not shortchange them.

CHAPTER 9

The Vaccination Ritual

> . . . at the cutting edge of scientific progress, where new ideas develop,
> we will never escape subjectivity; at a single point in time, we will all
> make our choices differently because of different insights and therefore
> different interpretations. Only the future will tell who was right.
>
> JAN P. VANDENBROUCKE
> "MEDICAL JOURNALS AND THE SHAPING OF MEDICAL KNOWLEDGE"
> LANCET, DECEMBER 19, 1998

Julie wrapped a towel around my freshly shampooed hair and led the way back to her station. I settled my very pregnant body as comfortably as possible on the chair. About three years before, we had discovered that we had a common interest in alternative medicine. These haircut appointments gave us ample time to swap stories and remedies.

"You're not vaccinating, are you?" Julie asked abruptly.

"Yes," I said, somewhat surprised. "Hannah's had all her shots, and I assume this baby will be immunized too." Being pregnant, I was eager to talk babies, but this subject wasn't on my agenda.

An uneasy silence settled between us. What was she thinking? Didn't she know the risk of leaving a child exposed to deadly diseases?

I suddenly felt defensive. "Why shouldn't my kids be vaccinated?"

Julie winced. "Because it's so hard on the immune system," she said. "It's just not very good to do."

My initial surprise transformed into disbelief and irritation. I wanted healthy children who were resistant to infectious diseases. Of *course* I was having them vaccinated. It was, I assumed, a way of guaranteeing that they would not fall victim to viruses like polio and measles.

"There are so many side effects from vaccines," added Julie.

Halfheartedly I asked if she knew of any literature about these supposed dangers of vaccines, but she couldn't refer me to any.

Well, one comment wasn't enough to rattle my convictions. A few months later when our second child arrived, we intended to follow the American Academy of Pediatrics's immunization schedule, with the exception of the newly recommended hepatitis B vaccine. Our seasoned pediatrician advised us to forego this one since he didn't perceive an epidemic and he didn't think our "clean living" warranted its use. So we waited two months to introduce our little bundle to the needle.

A month after Elle received her first DPT (diptheria, pertussis, tetanus) shot, we decided that Gregg's homeopath would be a good family doctor. I brought the girls in for their initial consultation. While taking their medical history, the doctor asked if they had been vaccinated. When I said that both children had received their immunizations on schedule, he expressed the same chagrin as Julie had.

"But where can I find some literature on vaccines?" I asked. He recently had moved from Denmark and was not yet familiar with the resources available in the United States. I wasn't familiar enough with the concepts of holistic health to dispense with one of our country's most fundamental rites of childhood. These were pre-

Internet days; I didn't know where to turn for information. I now knew two people vehemently opposed to vaccines. I wondered how many more people felt this way. I resisted the urge to seek more information. It was easier to follow majority opinion than face the possibility of controversy.

What finally set me on the path of enlightenment was the 1994 spring issue of *Mothering* magazine with its front cover headline "Are Vaccines Effective?" What I read about the tetanus vaccine in the corresponding story by Neil Miller made me stagger in the bookstore.

> In the wake of severe reaction to the original tetanus vaccine, the preparation was significantly diluted—some say to the point of clinical ineffectiveness. Nevertheless, vaccine-related complications persisted, including high fever, inner ear nerve damage, demyelinating neuropathy (a degenerative condition of the nervous system), anaphylactic shock, and loss of consciousness.[1]

Demyelinating neuropathy? Did I really read those words? Conventional medicine described my husband Gregg's condition as a demyelinating asymmetrical peripheral neuropathy. My mind jumped back ten years to 1985, the summer when he cut the bottom of his foot on a nail, went in for stitches, and received a routine tetanus shot. The tingling in his fingertips began about a year later. I knew it would be ever-so-unscientific to attribute the cause of his neuropathy to a tetanus vaccine; one could only hypothesize that a dose of tetanus toxoid might be a factor. It was a hypothesis, however, that I felt compelled to consider seriously.

This made me angry. The need to confront the whole darn issue irritated me. Why did vaccinations—the designated armor against childhood disease—have to be the topic of investigation, the point of rebellion? Why couldn't I be politically correct on this one? I just wanted to be a thirty-something mother worrying about how to get her toddler to sleep and when to start her baby on cereal. I didn't want to question this rite of passage. I didn't want to buck the medical infrastructure. What if I discovered that the negatives were significant enough to warrant a decision not to vaccinate? My pediatrician would holler at me; the schools would suspend my children—and I was not of the temperament to homeschool. What if I chose not to vaccinate and one of my daughters contracted a deadly disease and suffered a disability or worse? The burden of a wrong decision would damage me for life, too.

Then I began to wonder who opposes vaccines—medical heretics and radicals or competent scientists? What if vaccines compromise healthy immune systems? What if they provoke chronic problems? What if unvaccinated children stay healthier? A shower of questions challenged what I had taken for granted: that vaccines unequivocally were in my children's best interest. Finally, I saw the scope of my ignorance. I was having my daughters injected with powerful solutions that I knew little about for diseases that I knew little about. Thus began my research into the vaccine controversy.

The Current State of Affairs

In the United States, the Advisory Committee on Immunization Practices, a division of the Centers for Disease Control and Prevention (CDC) in Atlanta, Georgia, convenes three times a year to set the country's immunization policy. The majority of health professionals believes the benefits of these vaccines outweigh the negatives. Powerful institutions like the American Medical Association, the American Academy of Pediatrics, the CDC, and the World Health Organization—as well as multibillion-dollar pharmaceutical companies—tout the miracles of immunizations. "Take five and immunize," says one campaign ad plastered on the side of a city bus. Even McDonald's has advertised the immunization schedule on pamphlets conveniently located near the condiments.

The widely accepted theory behind immunization is that a half-milliliter of vaccine solution containing the weakened or killed virus or bacteria of a particular disease tricks the body into producing antibodies against that disease and, as a result, confers lifelong immunity. As populations build immunity, the disease in question will appear less and less frequently, to the point of extinction. This is the theory behind the disappearance of smallpox, officially declared eradicated on May 8, 1980. Scientists hope to add polio to this list of conquered diseases by the year 2005, and if the measles virus cooperates, by 2010 it too shall be declared a nuisance of the past.[2]

Through President Clinton's Childhood Immunization Initiative and a $500 million budget, a computer networking system is now available in some states to track a child's vaccination history through a Social Security number. This allows doctors to catch more opportunities to vaccinate. Even medical journals have jumped on the bandwagon with articles examining ways to increase the immunization rate. Whether constitutionally correct or not, some cities link vaccinations to welfare programs. In Dallas, Chicago, and New York, for instance, recipients of the Special Supplemental Nutrition Program for Women, Infants, and Children must have their children immunized before receiving benefits.[3]

So Where's the Controversy?

Without a doubt, vaccines sit high on the medical pedestal. We praise them for keeping us safe from infectious diseases. Occasionally, a vaccine fails in its mission. The rotavirus vaccine was licensed in 1998, but recalled in October 1999 after it caused bowel obstruction within weeks in a number of infants who had received it. Such a failure barely dents our positive perception of vaccines.

This current myopic vision prevents us from seeing the darker side of vaccinations. We almost need a supersensitive divining rod to detect it. After all, pediatricians' waiting rooms don't advertise books like Harris Coulter and Barbara Loe Fisher's *DPT: A Shot in the Dark* or Dr. Viera Scheibner's *Vaccination: The Medical Assault on the Immune System*. These writings, among many others, present vaccines in a far less heroic light. What is cause for great concern is that the currently obscure arguments against vaccines are well documented. Scheibner, for instance, based her conclusions on over thirty-five thousand medical documents, yet her work remains virtually unknown in mainstream medicine. She and other experts petition parents to consider carefully whether vaccinations are truly in their children's best interest. What's more, they urge the powers that be to rethink our country's vaccine program. Unfortunately, their cogent arguments tend to fall on deaf ears and closed minds.

One example of the medical establishment's unwillingness to acknowledge vaccine dangers occurred in 1982 when NBC aired "DPT: Vaccine Roulette," an Emmy award–winning documentary produced and hosted by the Washington D.C. reporter Lea Thompson. As it has done throughout history, the medical community refuted the claim that vaccines harm more than a negligible number of people. The *Journal of the American Medical Association* summed up the pervasive medical opinion in these words:

"Officially acknowledged experts on pertussis and DPT describe the NBC presentation as 'the most frightening bit of show business journalism I've ever seen,' 'biased, histrionic, and inaccurate,' and even 'amoral and psychopathic.'"[4]

Consumers, however, responded far differently. The show united parents of vaccine-damaged children. They formed the group Dissatisfied Parents Together (DPT), which now operates the National Vaccine Information Center (NVIC), whose primary purpose is to "prevent vaccine injuries and deaths through public education."[5] One of its toughest pupils has been Congress. It took five years of schooling before the National Childhood Vaccine Injury Act of 1986 was passed, setting up the first federal compensation program for vaccine-injured children on October 1, 1988. Unfortunately, this program has not operated as the NVIC had originally hoped it would. Because the Vaccine Injury Table so narrowly defines what constitutes a vaccine injury, few claims are paid. The program also protects vaccine manufacturers by making it illegal for vaccine-injured individuals to sue.

HISTORY'S HIDDEN SIDE

Almost since their inception, vaccines have had their share of problems. The English scientist and physician Edward Jenner is credited with creating vaccines during the late eighteenth century. While a medical student, Jenner was told by a milkmaid, "I cannot take smallpox for I have had cowpox."[6] Despite the fact that such statements were usually thought to be folklore, Jenner began to seriously consider this possibility. On May 14, 1796, he injected a healthy eight-year-old boy with the cowpox virus. Two years later, after vaccinating others, Jenner declared that the cowpox virus permanently protected against smallpox. In 1808, Parliament appropriated funds for the National Vaccine Establishment, which in turn launched mass immunization campaigns.

Louis Pasteur followed in Jenner's wake. He fueled the vaccine movement by developing the rabies vaccine and, more important, the germ theory. During the next 150 years, a plethora of scientists and researchers contributed to the world of vaccines. If you don a pair of rose-colored glasses, you might summarize the time line by saying that vaccines have grown safer and more effective and that, as a result, our children no longer contend with the symptoms of smallpox, the devastation of polio, or the misery of measles, among other diseases. The history of vaccinations looks about as creamy as a pint of Ben & Jerry's Cherry Garcia.

Peer beneath history's creamy veneer, however, and you'll find more than a handful of moldy cherries. For example, in 1928, an English physician named L. A. Parry wrote an article published in the *British Medical Journal*. Much to the horror of his colleagues, he expressed reservations about the smallpox vaccine. He noted that smallpox is five times as likely to be fatal in the vaccinated as in the unvaccinated. In 1870 about 85 percent of people were vaccinated, versus about 40 percent in 1925. Yet the years of least vaccination were the years of the fewest smallpox cases and the lowest mortality due to smallpox. He also pointed out that in areas with the highest vaccination rates—like Bombay and Calcutta—smallpox was still rampant, while in unvaccinated towns—like Leicester, England—it was almost unknown. Furthermore, 80 percent of patients admitted into the smallpox hospitals had been vaccinated, while only 20 percent had not.

Although Dr. Parry quoted facts and statistics in his article, his colleagues responded with this comment:

"We think that Dr. Parry, in his desire for enlightenment, would have been wiser not to introduce assumptions of fact into the framework of his questions."[7]

In 1979 the United States finally discontinued the smallpox vaccine amidst grumbling from the medical community. At the time, George Hardy, assistant director for the CDC, admitted, "There are effects of smallpox vaccine that are negative . . . it took more years than I would have thought was appropriate to reach a decision to stop using smallpox vaccine, but that happened."[8] His statement raises the question of just how appropriate other vaccine decisions have been during the past two decades.

THAT WAS THEN, WHAT ABOUT NOW?

But smallpox is gone, people argue. Sure, vaccines have some side effects and sometimes fail to work; even allopathic medicine acknowledges these drawbacks. No vaccine, admits many a medical article, is 100 percent safe or effective. Don't the benefits far outweigh the negatives? Isn't the picture better than it was?

True, the picture is different, but different is not always better. Instead of quarantine signs, we now have Ronald McDonald Houses for children with cancer and Make-A-Wish Foundations for terminally ill children. At the First International Public Conference on Vaccination, held in Alexandria, Virginia, in September 1997, speaker after speaker noted the changes in childhood diseases. Although the death rate of children under age fifteen has declined since 1900, the number of chronically disabled children doubled between 1982 and 1993. In the past two decades, asthma rates in the United States have increased by 75 percent. Allergies and autoimmune disorders also doubled between these years. In addition, autism, learning disabilities, and behavioral problems in children increased significantly.[9]

Is it mere coincidence that the appearance of these disorders follows the inception of mass immunization programs? Could vaccinations be silent contributors to these problems? A surprising number of scientists believe the latter. When you examine some facts and figures about the ten recommended immunizations, it's easier to understand why increasing numbers of physicians, researchers, parents, and others opt not to partake of our "mandatory" vaccination ritual.

TRIPLE ANTIGEN: PERTUSSIS, DIPHTHERIA, AND TETANUS

Pertussis

My aunt Pat, who is in her midseventies, had whooping cough in the early 1930s, but not nearly as bad as the children who lived behind her. "I could hear them coughing and coughing while they played in their backyard. I swore they turned inside out," she said.

Pertussis, commonly known as whooping cough or the "hundred-day cough," is a bacterial infection that typically begins as a cold, followed by an occasional cough. After about two weeks, such thick mucus develops that after being besieged by a violent coughing bout the child emits the trademark "whoop" as she gasps for air. This stage typically lasts anywhere from two to six weeks. Because whooping cough is often misdiagnosed, a special culture, which is still not completely accurate, must be taken to differentiate it from acute illnesses like bronchitis. According to Dr. Dorothy Shepherd, author of *Homeopathy in Epidemic Diseases,* pertussis responds well to homeopathic treatment.[10]

Since homeopathy had been suppressed by the time Aunt Pat was a child, about the only option available was to let the disease run its course. Fortunately, from 1900 to 1935 the number of deaths from pertussis declined by 79 percent in the United States and 82 percent in England.[11] The whole-cell pertussis vaccine, developed in the late 1930s, did not become nonmandatory protocol until the early 1940s.

The whole-cell pertussis vaccine was used until 1998, when the American Academy of Pediatrics decided to recommend the acellular (aP) version developed in 1981. This new version causes fewer adverse reactions. With the whole-cell pertussis vaccine, approximately half of recipients experienced pain at the injection site, fever over 100.4 degrees, and fretfulness.[12] One out of a hundred vaccine doses resulted in persistent crying (sometimes high-pitched screaming) lasting more than three hours. One out of 330 doses resulted in fevers greater than 104.5 degrees. One out of 1,750 doses resulted in seizures.[13] In addition, the whole-cell vaccine was linked, but not always by definitive scientific proof, to serious conditions like permanent neurological damage, brain damage, hyperactivity, attention deficit disorder, learning disabilities, autism, sudden infant death syndrome, and death. The list leaves one whooping.

Many people questioned not only the vaccine's safety, but also its efficacy. One of the numerous instances of properly vaccinated individuals catching pertussis occurred in Nova Scotia in 1987. Viera Scheibner reports on the study as follows:

> During the 28 months of enhanced surveillance, 526 cases of pertussis were identified (74/100,000 population). Most (91 percent) patients had received at least three doses of pertussis vaccine.
>
> By supplementing culture techniques with immunofluorescent staining and serological methods, they increased the laboratory confirmation from 17 percent to 65 percent, suggesting that strict clinical criteria accurately reflect the incidence.[Note: Pertussis cannot be diagnosed with 100 percent accuracy.] The authors concluded that pertussis remains a significant health problem in Nova Scotia despite nearly universal vaccination.[14]

Western Europe acknowledged the problems with the pertussis vaccine long before the United States. In 1976 West Germany stopped using the vaccine. Sweden followed suit in 1979, even though the country recorded nineteen thousand cases of pertussis between 1977 and 1979. But note: not one child died.[15] Japan also changed tactics. In 1975 the country suspended the use of the whole-cell vaccine when several children died after receiving it. After a short period, it was reinstated for use in children aged two and over. The acellular vaccine replaced it in 1981 and has been used ever since for all children, including infants. After conducting its own studies, Sweden still rejected the acellular pertussis vaccine.

The acellular vaccine is now protocol in the United States. Before we get complacent and think our babies are completely safe, know that the same adverse reactions have been reported following the use of this vaccine, albeit with less frequency, and are still under investigation. The journal *Pediatric Annals* reported in June 1997 that "because more severe reaction (e.g., anaphylaxis, encephalopathy) occur so rarely, postlicensure surveillance will be required to evaluate these reactions after DTaP vaccines."[16]

Diphtheria

In the early 1900s Eleanor Walsh suffered a massive heartbreak. Within two months, her three oldest children, all under the age of seven, died from diphtheria. Just the thought of her plight would make any mother's heart ache. Fortunately, diphtheria no longer affects child mortality statistics in the United States, but it is still a problem in developing countries whose sanitation efforts fall well below our accepted norm.

Like pertussis, diphtheria is a bacterial disease. Symptoms include a sore throat, fever, and wheezing. As the disease worsens, a membrane may cover the throat and tonsils, making breathing difficult to the point of suffocation. No wonder diphtheria was dreaded in the late nineteenth and early twentieth centuries, when it was at its height.

Most of its victims were children between the ages of two and five.

In 1900 diphtheria claimed the lives of nine hundred of every million children.[17] Between 1900 and 1920 the mortality rate declined by 50 percent.[18] The diphtheria toxoid vaccine was not invented until 1926, and national immunization did not begin until 1942.

Although the diphtheria toxoid vaccine has been credited with saving many lives, lapses in its efficacy have occurred. For example, in a 1969 outbreak in Chicago, 37.5 percent of diptheria victims had been fully vaccinated or showed medical evidence of full immunity. A report on another outbreak revealed that 61 percent of the total cases and 33 percent of the fatal cases had been fully vaccinated.[19]

The fact that no diptheria cases were reported in the United States in 1995 obscures such examples of a questionable vaccine.[20] It's too bad that nobody knows the long-term effects of the diphtheria toxoid vaccine. Most important, we cannot determine definitively how better sanitation and nutrition have influenced diphtheria's decline. Since this disease still plagues third-world countries, you would think that sanitation and nutrition play a significant role in its progression—and the progression of other infectious diseases. Perhaps the role of hygiene deserves its fifteen minutes of fame.

Tetanus

When my daughters were still quite young, we moved into a subdivision under construction. For the next two years I constantly admonished them to watch out for nails. The corner bus stop alone boasted enough to build a garage.

The possibility of a child suffering a puncture wound and developing tetanus is a fear that most parents harbor. We need to remember, however, that the tetanus bacterium thrives in soil and animal manure and can only survive in a bodily wound if the wound is free of oxygen. Thus, thorough wound cleansing is the best way to prevent tetanus.

Tetanus remains difficult to treat. Symptoms of the disease can progress from muscle stiffness to muscle rigidity so intense that bones fracture and respiration stops. Despite this gruesome scenario, the pros and cons of the tetanus vaccine should still be weighed. Since 1976, fewer than one hundred cases of tetanus have occurred in the United States. On average, less than 5 percent of cases occur in people under age fifty, and of this 5 percent the case fatality rate is less than 5 percent.[21]

The tetanus vaccine has been linked to chronic central nervous system disorders including multiple sclerosis, peripheral neuropathies, Guillain-Barré syndrome, and arthritis.[22] Long-term adverse effects are very difficult to study, because tetanus toxoid is usually administered in conjunction with the diphtheria toxoid and pertussis vaccines. One question to consider is whether it is worth risking these adverse reactions when so few cases of tetanus occur.

In his most recent book, *The Vaccine Guide: Making An Informed Choice*, Dr. Randall Neustaedter presents parents with two options. One is to delay the vaccine until a child is twelve months old, since infants who cannot walk are at an extremely low risk for the type of wound that causes tetanus. The second option is to skip the vaccine and use tetanus immune globulin (TIG) in the event of injury.[23] This is a human blood product that is said to provide immunity for twenty-eight days.[24] It can be used immediately after an injury occurs.

My friend Laura chose to use TIG when her daughter Sasha burned her hand and the wound became infected. When Laura resisted using the tetanus vaccine, the emergency room doctor suggested TIG. Sasha recovered normally and Laura found some peace of mind without having to introduce a vaccine into her child's body.

ANOTHER 3-IN-1: MEASLES, MUMPS, AND RUBELLA

Measles

"Auntie Em took care of me when I had the measles," Dorothy says in *The Wizard of Oz*. If you watch this classic, you can't help but wonder if today's children will grow up perceiving measles as a killer disease. It can be argued that we have taken to vaccinating against diseases that are more of a nuisance than they are a danger.

In his book *How to Raise a Healthy Child . . . in Spite of Your Doctor,* Dr. Robert Mendelsohn maintains that "no treatment is required for measles" except for bed rest, fluids, and perhaps a darkened room to alleviate eye irritation.[25] Chinese medicine views measles as "a beneficial disease that rids the body of accumulated poisons. After suffering this illness, parents will notice a change in a child's behavior, attitude, and attention. Most likely, a child will be less irritable, less negative, and healthier."[26] This does not mean that a child will not feel ill. A barking cough, itchy eyes, maybe a sore throat, a runny nose, and a fever as high as 105 degrees tend to zap the energy right out of busy bodies.

Although homeopathy and Ayurveda treat measles efficiently and effectively, the medical world chose to meet measles head-on with a live virus vaccine introduced in 1963. However, the disease had already declined naturally—by a whopping 95 percent from its peak year in 1941.[27] The case load continued to decrease after the introduction of the measles vaccine and in 1978, the United States announced a goal to eradicate measles by 1981.

But measles entered the decade like a lion, not a lamb. Suddenly the disease was on the rise again. In 1985 the federal government reported 1,984 nonpreventable cases of measles, 80 percent of which occurred in vaccinated individuals.[28] In 1992 a spokesperson for the Ohio Department of Health told the *Dayton Daily News* that 2,720 cases of measles were reported in Ohio during 1989. "Get shots or forget the seventh grade," the spokesperson warned. But what he failed to mention, reports Dr. Kristine Severyn—founder of Ohio Parents for Vaccine Safety, now called the Vaccine Policy Institute—is that more than 72 percent of these cases were in vaccinated people.

The list of adverse reactions associated with the measles vaccine is long. Encephalopathy (a degenerative condition of the brain), neurological disorders, mental retardation, aseptic meningitis, and seizure disorders are listed as primary complications. Secondary complications include Reye's syndrome, Guillain-Barré syndrome, blood clotting disorders, juvenile-onset diabetes, and Hodgkin's disease.[29] In 1995 the *Lancet* reported that those who receive the measles vaccine are three times more likely to develop Crohn's disease and more than twice as likely to develop ulcerative colitis.[30] With all these potential problems, why does conventional medicine claim that the measles vaccine, not to mention other vaccines, is highly safe and effective?

Mumps

In 1970, at the age of nine, Debbie contracted mumps. She remembers having the characteristic chipmunk cheeks and staying home from school for a week. She says that looking at herself in the mirror caused more pain than swallowing. Jennifer also remembers mumps. Her memory is of receiving special attention, which, as a middle child, she relished.

Dr. Mendelsohn calls mumps "an innocuous disease" that does not require medical treatment. Mumps is a viral disease said to be spread by coughing, sneezing, or just breathing the air near someone who is infected. Mumps may be innocuous, but it can also be painful because the disease affects the salivary gland. Pain in swallowing, a fever ranging from 100 to 104 degrees, no appetite, a sore back, and headaches can make for a miserable darling.

Mumps rarely results in death, however, and severe complications are more common in individuals over age twenty. The most serious concern is that an adult male who was mumps free as a child contracts the illness and develops orchitis. This is a disease of the testicles that can result in sterility, but sterility in both testicles is rare.

So why is there a mumps vaccine? That's a good question. Dr. Mendelsohn writes:

> If the mumps immunization is given to protect adult males from orchitis, not to prevent children from getting mumps, it would seem reasonable to administer it only to those males who haven't developed natural immunity by the time they reach puberty. They would then be more certain of protection as adults. All girls and countless boys would avoid the potential consequences of a hazardous vaccine.[31]

The long-term side effects of this immunization are unknown. The mumps vaccine has been associated with complications similar to that of measles: fevers, seizures, encephalitis, and severe atypical mumps disease. One study contends that women who have had mumps in childhood are less likely to get ovarian cancer.[32] Once the vaccine became part of mass immunization campaigns, mumps started afflicting more adolescents and adults, both of whom suffer more severe symptoms and complications.

Rubella

Dr. Benjamin Spock calls rubella "a relatively harmless disease."[33] Like measles and mumps, this virus—commonly called German measles or "the three-day rash"—is cyclical, with increases every six to nine years, mostly in winter and spring. If your child develops rubella, he may have a fever, sore throat, cold symptoms, and a rash that first appears on the face and scalp and then spreads to the arms and body. This rash usually disappears within two to three days. No treatment is recommended. Rarely do side effects occur, although brain inflammation and chronic arthritis are possible complications.[34]

The main concern regarding rubella is pregnant women in their first trimester who have contracted the disease for the first time. Between 20 and 50 percent of babies born to these moms will have birth defects.[35] The reason children are vaccinated for rubella is not because of the horrible side effects of the disease itself, but to prevent pregnant women who have not had the illness from getting it.

This sounds like a very noble cause, except that the vaccine is not free of side effects. It has been linked to chronic fatigue syndrome, acute arthritis, chronic persistent arthritis, central and peripheral nervous system disorders, Guillain-Barré syndrome, and thrombocytopenia, which involves a decrease in blood platelets, resulting in spontaneous bleeding. [36]

In September 1997, the newsletter from Ohio Parents for Vaccine Safety related the story of Dr. Joanne Hatem:

> Dr. Hatem was a victim of rubella vaccine administered as a requirement for a medical residency in New York State. As a consequence of the rubella vaccine, Dr. Hatem was left with chronic rubella viremia, afflicting her with chronic arthritis, chronic fatigue, and other physical ailments, causing her to give up her gastroenterology practice. Dr. Hatem was a brilliant woman, who spent several years combing the federal government records for rubella vaccine licensing procedures. As a result, she discovered that the currently used rubella vaccine was inadequately tested in adult females prior to U.S. licensing, even

though it is routinely administered to adult females. Rubella vaccine adverse reactions occur at much higher rates in adult females, as compared to children and men.[37]

Dr. Hatem died on September 6, 1997, from complications that she believed were caused by the rubella vaccine. Extrapolate this scenario into the world of children. Can we trust that the testing of the rubella vaccine, as well as all other vaccines, is more than adequate for our children? Or are our babies, toddlers, preschoolers, and even adolescents innocent guinea pigs in our quest to conquer disease?

POLIO

Anne chose not to vaccinate her two children. "Not even for polio?" her friend Patricia tentatively asked. "That's the one that scares me the most." For many a baby boomer, this fear grips hard; the epidemic of the 1950s still haunts us. It's a difficult memory to erase, especially when most of us know someone who walks with a limp due to the ravages of polio.

Polio has existed for centuries. A 1932 article in the *Journal of the American Medical Association* described the nature of this viral disease as seasonal. The authors also stated that "because clinical cases of polio are numerically far too few they cannot account for the universal natural immunity of the adult population."[38] Back then, it was seen as a disease of infancy, with about 90 percent of infected children and adults recovering normally. In fact, the natural polio virus produces no symptoms at all in over 90 percent of those exposed to it, even under epidemic conditions.[39]

As we all know, polio can cripple individuals, as it did President Franklin Delano Roosevelt, who contracted the disease at age thirty-nine. The polio vaccine, developed by Jonas Salk, was introduced amidst great hoopla on April 12, 1955, the tenth anniversary of Roosevelt's death. This killed-virus vaccine was praised as a "safe, potent, and efficient" prevention for polio. Two months later, tragedy struck Denver. The American Public Health Service confirmed that 168 cases of poliomyelitis had developed in vaccinated children. Six of these children died. Another 149 unvaccinated children contracted the disease from vaccinated children who had never suffered the disease; another six children died.[40]

Other reports of outbreaks following mass immunization caused the United States to rethink its tactics. In 1966 the government officially switched to the Sabin vaccine. This live-virus version was simpler to administer since it was taken orally and was reported to be more effective with fewer side effects. Nevertheless, an underground debate continued regarding which vaccine was truly better and safer—the inactivated polio vaccine (IPV) or the oral polio vaccine (OPV). The pendulum again swung in January 2000. Because all polio cases since 1979 are believed to have been OPV induced, the Advisory Committee of Immunization Practices (ACIP) now recommends using the IPV for all doses. This inactivated vaccine cannot transmit the disease from a vaccinated person to another person.

THE NEW SHOTS ON THE BLOCK

Hepatitis B

The birth of Yvonne and Rick Wilson's first child in 1991 coincided with the first recommendation of the hepatitis B vaccine for all infants. It wasn't until a few years later when the Wilsons started looking into vaccines that they realized what a great favor their pediatrician had done for them in 1991. Based on the Wilsons' clean lifestyle and medical history, Dr. Thompson reasoned that their baby didn't need a hepatitis B vaccine. In retrospect, the Wilsons were relieved that someone was thinking, because they had not given the subject a nanosecond of thought.

So, let's think about it now. First of all, hepatitis B falls into the category of adult diseases, not infectious childhood diseases like measles and mumps. In fact, it is considered a sexually transmitted disease. Individuals at high risk include prostitutes, sexually active homosexual males, intravenous drug users, people exposed to blood contaminated with the virus, and babies born to infected mothers.

According to the National Vaccine Information Center:

In 1992, there were 16,126 cases of hepatitis B reported in the U.S. with 903 deaths attributed to either chronic infection or complications from an acute infection. In 1994, there were 12,517 cases reported and the Centers for Disease Control stated that "hepatitis B continues to decline in most states, primarily because of changes in high-risk behaviors among injecting-drug users."[41]

So why does the ACIP recommend that all babies be vaccinated, even those born to parents who abstain from drugs and live in clean homes and neighborhoods? Dr. George Peter, chairman of the American Academy of Pediatrics, shed some light on this question in 1992. First, he said, hepatitis B remains a public health problem that sometimes occurs outside of high-risk groups. Second, high-risk groups don't seek out the vaccine and are difficult to reach. Third, babies are accessible. Fourth, it is cheaper to vaccinate an 8-pound infant than a 150-pound adult, since less vaccine solution is needed.[42] Is this how we want our children and babies used in the fight against disease?

Unfortunately, the vaccine has a list of "unknowns" attached to it. No one fully understands the intricacies of the newborn immune system, so no one can say for sure how the vaccine affects this system. Although the duration of vaccine immunity is estimated to be about thirteen years, studies continue in this area. Other studies link the vaccine to neurological disorders such as demyelinating diseases, autoimmune disorders, Guillain-Barré syndrome, and multiple sclerosis.[43]

It isn't reassuring to know that "following the CDC recommendation in 1991 that all infants receive hepatitis vaccine, only 32 percent of pediatricians in North Carolina responding to a survey questionnaire thought the vaccine was warranted for all newborns." [44]

Immunologist Burton Waisbren, M.D., points out that a blood test can determine if a mother is a hepatitis B carrier. Rather than vaccinating all newborns, he suggests that hospitals mandate this blood test before a mother delivers. In Wisconsin, where Dr. Waisbren practices, only one case of hepatitis B in a child under ten years of age occurred in the past ten years.[45] Dr. Waisbren advocates that a moratorium be placed on the universal hepatitis B vaccination program.[46]

HiB (*Haemophilus influenzae* Type B Meningitis)

Talia's mother, Karen, didn't intend to vaccinate her baby at all, but the pediatrician talked her into immunizing for the *Haemophilus influenzae* type B bacteria. The infection, he warned, is difficult to diagnose because the symptoms mimic the flu, and meningitis and pneumonia are possible complications. Karen thought this sounded scary, so she agreed. It's a challenge for a mother not to be emotionally vulnerable. The second the needle went into her nine-month-old's little arm, she instinctively knew it was the wrong decision. Within two hours, Talia's fever soared and any movement set her to screaming. Karen's late-night calls to the clinic were answered with the pat statement, "This reaction is normal. Don't worry." But Karen didn't think it was normal, even though Talia did not appear to suffer from any long-term side effects.

Along with tetanus and polio, meningitis is a dreaded disease. The odds of contracting Hib are far less in the first twelve to eighteen months if a mother breast-feeds her infant. If you recall from previous chapters, the role of maternal antibodies in protecting an infant and helping his immune system develop cannot be overstated. Some studies show that a child's risk for Hib is lower if he does not attend day care. In one study conducted in 1986, "50 percent of all invasive disease caused by *H. influenzae* type B was attributable to day care settings."[47]

In 1995, 1,164 cases of Hib occurred. The disease probably peaked in the mid-1980s, although the incidence of Hib during that time was not officially recorded. It is thought to have occurred more frequently in the '70s and '80s than it did in the '90s. Randall Neustaedter points out an interesting observation that is reiterated by other authors:

> Some observers associate this increase with the administration of other vaccines and their apparent ability to impair immune system resistance. Although this link has not been proven the tendency of vaccines to cause neurological complications has raised suspicion that central nervous system infections occur more frequently as a direct result of DTP and measles vaccine.[48]

In other words, routine vaccinations may have encouraged the spread of diseases like Hib.

Even though the cases of Hib have decreased in the past decade, at what price has this occurred? The Hib vaccine is not free of dangers; on the contrary, it is associated with an increased incidence of the disease following vaccination. Many of the same disorders mentioned before—central nervous system diseases, Guillain-Barré syndrome, and seizures—appear with HiB as well, in addition to thrombocytopenia purpura, a condition where blood seeps spontaneously from vessels due to a decrease in blood platelets.[49]

Chicken Pox

Within a day of getting chicken pox, four-year-old Hannah declared, "Chicken pox are not fun." Fortunately, her fever and itchies disappeared after seventy-two hours. That's not so bad when compared with Mary and M.J., who both contracted chicken pox as adults. They were miserable for a solid week, which is no fun when young children are underfoot.

According to the CDC, prior to the vaccine, approximately 3.7 million cases of varicella zoster virus—or chicken pox—occurred annually in the United States and resulted in about one hundred deaths. Most of these deaths occurred as a result of secondary infections, particularly strep infections.[50] Concern over preventing deaths in children and adults prompted researchers to develop a vaccine for chicken pox. It's costly, however, for pharmaceutical companies to develop a vaccine and not offer it to the entire population. In addition, when the annual cost of chicken pox is estimated at $400 million—95 percent of which is wages lost by parents who must miss work in order to care for their sick children—the vaccine sounds helpful, especially when it is billed as safe and effective.[51] So on March 17, 1995, the FDA approved Varivax, the shot intended to wipe out the pesky pox from the general population.

Media campaigns effectively continue to perpetuate fears about this disease. One vaccine advertisement in a medical journal had a photo of a young girl. Her face was puffy, swollen, and bright red, almost to the point of being grotesque. Any caring doctor viewing this ad would understandably be inclined to push the vaccine's use. Health care professionals are influenced not only by the worst-case scenarios they treat, but also by the advertising promotions of vaccine manufacturers.

In *The Consumer's Guide to Childhood Vaccines,* author Barbara Loe Fisher points out that the varicella zoster vaccine manufacturer states in the product insert that "the vaccine has not been evaluated for its carcinogenic or mutagenic potential, or its potential to impair fertility." Furthermore, the insert states, "There are no data relating to simultaneous administration of [the vaccine] with DTP or DPV."[52] Proponents of the vaccine claim that it has been safely used for almost twenty years, but if the vaccine's potential to cause cancer or infertility has not been studied, how accurate is this claim?

ARTIFICIAL VS. NATURAL IMMUNITY

One other point concerning vaccines demands attention. It pertains to how we acquire immunity. When my daughter Hannah received her first MMR (measles, mumps, rubella) shot, the antigens in the vaccine directly entered her muscle and bloodstream. Just as the pediatrician warned, in about ten days her fever spiked to 103 degrees and she developed diarrhea. Supposedly she now has immunity to measles, mumps, and rubella. Her immunity is artificially induced versus naturally induced.

When immunity develops naturally, viruses enter the body through the nose, mouth, or skin. Many measles cases don't develop because the host sneezes them away. Vaccines, on the other hand, bypass these natural protective ports of entry and quickly gain entry into the major organs and tissues. In 1996 *Pediatrics Journal* confirmed that "we are getting better at tricking the body" with vaccines.[53] What exactly happens to the toxins that are injected into the still-developing immune systems of infants and children? They can't sneeze away an injection.

At this point, no one can say for certain what happens. By the time a child is eighteen months old, he will have been injected with over thirty doses of antigens, all of which will have entered the body unnaturally. Short-term reactions to this barrage of bacteria, viruses, and preservatives—like formalin and thimerosal (derivatives of the carcinogens formaldehyde and mercury, respectively)—are unpredictable. If a child develops cancer, a brain tumor, ADD, allergies, eczema, asthma, recurrent ear infections, or bronchitis, no one will be able to determine if a vaccination played a part. Scientists know how to create vaccines; they know far, far less about how these toxins assault the immune system or other body parts over a lifetime. Dr. Richard Moskowitz suggests that we eliminate the term *immunization* from our vocabulary. Who can say for sure that vaccines safely and effectively induce immunity when substantial evidence indicates that they weaken immune systems?

In her book *Vaccination: The Medical Assault on the Immune System*, scientist Viera Scheibner addresses the vaccine problem:

> Various elements of vaccines can stay in the body for long periods of time, some of them permanently, often by incorporating themselves into the genetic material of the host's cells. This provokes constant effort to expel these foreign substances leading to a systematic weakening of the immune system. Constant antigenic stimulation of the immune system leads to cancer and leukemia and a host of other autoimmune diseases.[54]

Instead of providing protection against acute infectious diseases, vaccination drives the disease deeper into the body and leads to chronic infestation by the pathogenic agent. Asthma, allergies, ADD, arthritis, multiple sclerosis, warts, herpes, shingles, and AIDS are examples of the chronic conditions that some scientists and medical experts believe result from vaccines.[55] The majority of the medical community, however, disagrees with this theory.

TO VACCINATE OR NOT TO VACCINATE

Weighing the pros and cons of vaccines may be one of the most difficult, confusing tasks that you will ever undertake. At times, you may feel absolutely certain that one side is correct. Then, upon reading an opposing opinion, you will find yourself leaning toward the other camp. Both sides can sling statistics at you all day and all night. Of course, these studies and statistics need to be considered. But if you peel away the layers of theories, what lies at the heart of the matter is your philosophical approach to health.

As Dr. Moskowitz says:

> Taking responsibility for not vaccinating is no different from taking responsibility for a home birth or any other form of alternative health care. It calls not for a substitute for conventional care, but rather a different relationship to the healing process and the health care system based on personal choice and direct participation.[56]

When you develop this different relationship with health—the holistic relationship that we have explored—foregoing vaccines is not only logical but also no longer frightening. Unfortunately, in our society this requires change for most of us.

If you choose not to vaccinate, know that your journey does not end. Lisa investigated the subject and relayed her findings to her spouse Steve. They both agreed that vaccinations did not seem to be in their baby's best interest. Cindy encountered much rockier waters when she suggested to her husband Robert that they evaluate vaccinating their children. It took considerable time and study before Robert concluded that they should stop vaccinating their child.

If you choose to tell your extended family of your decision to abstain, be prepared for a reaction ranging from furrowed brows to an outcry of "Do you want to kill your kids?" Whatever the response, hold your ground. You are the one who has researched the issue, debated it, listened to your gut feeling, and had the courage to choose.

Dealing with your doctor can elicit just as varied a response. Suzanne never had a doctor reprimand her, pressure her, or threaten her for choosing to forgo vaccinations. All were respectful of her decision. One suggested that she might want to rethink the tetanus vaccine, but she just said, "No, thank you." Horror stories, however, abound. Ellen had to contend with an emergency room doctor who, upon discovering that he was tending to an unvaccinated child, was more concerned about giving little Alex her shots than treating her acute illness. Ellen held her ground. Beth, on the other hand, decided she didn't want her newborn vaccinated for hepatitis B. This made her husband and doctor very nervous. In fact, the pediatrician phoned her two days after she took her baby home and pressured her, saying that she was a bad mother and endangering her child. Still emotional from the birth experience, Beth finally caved in. She said she felt literally sick to her stomach when her baby was vaccinated. Remember that you aren't tied to your doctor for life. Children survive when they change cities and schools. They will certainly survive if you change pediatricians.

If you decide to vaccinate, the National Vaccine Information Center suggests that you ask these eight questions before you proceed:

1. Is my child sick right now?
2. Has my child had a bad reaction to a vaccination before?
3. Does my child have a personal or family history of:

- vaccine reactions?
- convulsions or neurological disorders?
- severe allergies?
- immune system disorders?

4. Do I know if my child is at high risk of reacting?
5. Do I have full information on the vaccine's side effects?
6. Do I know how to identify a vaccine reaction?
7. Do I know how to report a vaccine reaction?
8. Do I know the vaccine manufacturer's name and lot number?[57]

No matter what you decide, if you believe that your decision is in your child's best interest, find the strength within you to uphold it.

VACCINE EXEMPTIONS

How can I sit tight, you say, when vaccines are mandatory? "Since the repeal of the draft in the 1970s, mandatory vaccination remains the only law that requires a citizen to risk his life for his country," say Harris Coulter and Barbara Loe Fisher in *A Shot in the Dark*.[58] Each state retains sovereignty over its vaccination laws. What most residents don't know is that every state offers at least one type of exemption from "mandatory" vaccination laws.

Currently, fifteen states allow a philosophical exemption from vaccination. All fifty states allow a medical exemption, and all states except Mississippi and West Virginia allow a religious exemption.[59]

If a philosophical exemption is not available, you can search for a physician or osteopath who is willing to discuss signing for a medical exemption. If you have a family history of allergies, asthma, or neurological disorders, you may want to seriously consider this option. Let your fingers do the walking through the yellow pages and you can probably find a professional who will honor your request.

You can also refer to the holistic publications in your area. Many health food stores and co-ops, metaphysical stores, and public libraries provide these newspapers and magazines free of charge. Contact the physicians who place advertisements in or write articles for such publications.

If you claim a religious exemption, expect extra legwork. Some states require specific wording for a religious exemption. It may be in your best interest to consult a library. Ask a librarian to help you find the state statutes so that you can make certain that if you need to write out the exemption, you know the correct language to use. You can also purchase a copy of *Your Personal Guide to Immunization Exemptions,* by Grace Girdwain, which includes samples of exemption letters. (See the resources section.)

THE FUTURE

For now, vaccines remain firmly lodged in our health care system. Scientists continuously work to develop new vaccinations for our health challenges including the common cold, cancers, and genital warts. Vaccines have already been developed and approved for Lyme disease and influenza. An AIDS vaccine and a birth control vaccine currently are being tested. There is even talk of the "supervaccine," the all-in-one shot to set your immunity for life. We seem to do everything within our scientific power and budget to avoid the slings and arrows of disease.

But life is neither all yin nor all yang. It is a combination. We cannot protect our children against death and grief. We cannot isolate them from the inhumanity of some humans. We cannot offer them a world free of disease. This would be to defy nature. It would be like giving our children a night sky always bestowed with bright stars and a full moon. Nature, we forget, has her own rhythms and cycles. Her intelligence is absolute, whereas ours is only learned. Many diseases are cyclical and keep coming back no matter how hard we try to eradicate them. We forget that they benefit us in the long run by strengthening our immune systems.

Let us hope that the United States will follow the lead of countries like Britain and Sweden and make vaccinations optional. The real change will happen when we accept a holistic framework of health and truly live within that framework. We have a long journey ahead. Let's just hope that our great-great-grandchildren don't look back and sadly say, "They knew not what they did."

CHAPTER 10

Open Wide: Holistic Dentistry

The truth is that every dental procedure is an invasion of the human
system and may generate an adverse response somewhere in the
human body.

MARK A. BEINER, D.D.S.
WHOLE-BODY DENTISTRY

The dentist slid my new blue toothbrush out of its box. He
wanted to make certain that I knew how to brush properly since
this was my first appointment with him. Being a captive audience,
I had no choice but to listen, even though at age thirty-four, with
only a few cavities in my dental history, I figured that my brushing
wasn't too far off the mark. Dr. Allen picked up a plastic bottle and
sprinkled a white powder onto the toothbrush bristles. From an
opaque bottle, he dribbled a clear liquid over the powder.

"This is all you need when you brush," he said. "A little baking
soda and hydrogen peroxide."

I'm sure that my eyebrows arched. Was he suggesting that I stop
buying toothpaste? That I forget about fluoride? Why, this method
negated the golden rule of dentistry that had been ingrained in me
since grade school: Fluoride fights cavities.

This was my first visit to a holistic dentist. It definitely had a
different flavor than my past experiences. Of course, Dr. Allen

examined and cleaned my teeth, examined my gums, and checked my bite and my tongue—all the things a proficient dentist normally does. But he also spent a good deal of time inquiring about my diet. How often did I eat? What foods did I favor? Did I eat a lot of sweets? How about fruits and vegetables? Were the foods organic? Did I drink milk? coffee? tea? soda? How much water did I consume each day? I felt as if I were visiting a nutritionist, not someone who specialized in teeth. Dr. Allen explained how a diet balanced in minerals and nutrients strengthens the teeth from the inside out. Proper food, he said, is the best prevention of tooth decay.

I have since had occasion to visit two other holistic dentists. The Environmental Dental Association estimates that 5 percent of all dentists licensed in the United States practice holistic dentistry, also called whole-body dentistry or biological dentistry. None of the dentists whom I saw recommended or offered a fluoride treatment. All three informed me of the potential toxicity of mercury fillings and handed me pertinent scientific literature. They said it was totally my choice whether I wanted to keep my fillings or replace them with a mercury-free material. In addition, one of the dentists used cranial sacral therapy to help align my bite. During a cranial sacral session, the practitioner gently presses on the skull bones, a most pleasant experience. I think it was the first time that I ever naturally relaxed in the dentist's chair. Some whole-body dentists also integrate therapies like homeopathy and acupuncture into their practice.

THE HEART OF HOLISTIC DENTISTRY

Although holistic dentists may use a variety of complementary therapies, they all recognize the relationship between the mouth and the body. They believe that what happens in the mouth positively or negatively influences the general health of the body. Dental infections, dental procedures such as root canals and fillings, and dental toxins like mercury and nickel may very well impact the body on some level, be it physically, emotionally, or even spiritually. Accordingly, a number of holistic dental organizations—including the International Academy of Oral Medicine and Toxicology and the American Academy of Biological Dentistry—advocate the use of nontoxic materials in dentistry.

As you now can understand, considering the mouth without considering the rest of the body contradicts the concept of holistic health practice. At first, it was difficult for me to think that a filling or a root canal could play a part in diseases like fibromyalgia, hypothyroidism, or Alzheimer's. Yet I've come to see that within a holistic paradigm, holistic dentistry makes perfect sense.

Beginning in the late 1940s, Dr. Reinhold Voll, a medical doctor, anatomy professor, and acupuncturist, began to map the energetic connections between teeth and organs. Over forty years, he diagramed a complex web of energy pathways that connects organs and teeth. For centuries, Traditional Chinese Medicine (TCM) has worked with pathways called meridians. Some of Voll's meridians correspond to the meridians of TCM, while others do not. For example, according to Voll's chart the second molar shares a meridian with the left mammary gland, the pancreas, the jaw, the thyroid, and the parathyroid.[1] If something goes haywire with the second molar, these organs could be affected, and vice versa. Today these charts are becoming more visible within the field of dentistry, although they are far from commonplace.

Holistic dentists and conventional dentists view issues from different perspectives. Two topics currently debated in all corners of the dental arena concern fluoride and amalgam fillings. Whether or not you visit a holistic dentist, these areas are worth exploring. They particularly pertain to the well-being of children, who tend to be much more sensitive than adults to the substances put in their bodies.

FLUORIDE

In April 1999, the *Toronto Star* quoted Dr. Hardy Limeback, professor of dentistry at the University of Toronto and oft-cited proponent of fluoride, as saying:

> Children under three should never use fluoridated toothpaste. Or drink fluoridated water. And baby formula must never be made up using Toronto tap water [which is fluoridated]. Never. In fluoridated areas, people should never use fluoride supplements. We tried to get them banned for children but [the dentists] wouldn't even look at the evidence we presented.[2]

The question that immediately came to my mind after reading this article was: What persuaded this pro-fluoride dentist to discourage giving fluoride in any form to young children and babies? When I compared his recommendation to that of the American Dental Association (ADA), I discovered a discrepancy. The ADA recommends fluoride for children between six months and three years. If water is not sufficiently fluoridated, this age group should take a .25-milligram fluoride supplement.[3] On average, fluoridated water contains .7 to 1.2 parts per million.

Even before Grand Rapids, Michigan, became the first community in the United States to fluoridate its public drinking water back in 1945, the ADA had advocated fluoride as a preventative health measure. The organization contends that scientific studies adequately prove that when fluoride is incorporated into tooth enamel, which is the protective coating on a tooth, the tooth better resists decay. Decay, it says, occurs when bacteria and plaque organisms release harmful acids. Fluoride ions in the enamel interfere with the release of these acids. The ions also help reverse the early stages of enamel decay. I never questioned this theory until I discovered that a notable number of dentists, researchers, politicians, and consumers oppose the use of fluoride in public drinking water, supplements, and even in toothpaste.

Before we address the controversy, let's review the indisputable facts about fluoride. First, it is a substance found in nature. Some places on Earth have very concentrated levels of naturally occurring fluoride, while other areas have next to none. Thus, humans have always been exposed to at least a trace of fluoride. Second, scientists agree that raw fluoride is poisonous—almost as poisonous as arsenic. Third, since 1931 the dental profession has recognized that too much fluoride in the body causes dental fluorosis, a disease that discolors the teeth. In severe cases, teeth turn brown; in mild cases they appear mottled with barely detectable to noticeable white spots. In areas where drinking water contains the optimal 1 part per million (ppm) of fluoride, about one-fifth of children develop mild fluorosis.[4] Fourth, in 1998 the FDA mandated that all products containing fluoride include a warning that fluoride is toxic to children. Fluoridated toothpaste contains one to two thousand times more fluoride than fluoridated water.[5] On the back of fluoridated toothpaste tubes, you will find the recommendation that children use a pea-sized amount of toothpaste so that less has a chance to be swallowed. If a child swallows a large amount of toothpaste, a call to the poison control center is in order.

Once we go beyond these facts, opinions diverge. The ADA states that fluoride prevents 40 to 60 percent of cavities for people living in fluoridated communities.[6] In addition, the ADA argues that no study has definitively shown that fluoride negatively impacts one's general health. Until proven otherwise, the ADA labels fluoride a safe substance, incapable of harming the body when ingested below certain limits. Most important, the organization contends that fluoride prevents tooth decay. Thus, fluoridated water and toothpaste, topical fluoride treatments, and fluoride supplements in nonfluoridated areas are in everyone's best interest. The only exception is the rare person who is allergic to fluoride.

Voices on the other side of the fence espouse the opposite. Although they agree that no study has shown unequivocally that low levels of fluoride damage the body, opponents of fluoridation maintain that a multitude of studies suggest that fluoride interferes with processes in the body. In his book *Fluoride the Aging Factor*, Dr. John Yiamouyiannis cites research from the United States, Japan, Poland, India, and Australia which indicates that fluoride disrupts the synthesis of collagen, a protein found in our skin, tendons, ligaments, muscles, and cartilage.[7] This protein also is necessary for calcium and phosphorous to create bone, tooth enamel, and dentin, the inner part of the tooth. Studies from Japan and Poland show that when as little as 1 ppm fluoride is added to the drinking water of lab animals, certain amino acids indicative of disrupted collagen synthesis appear in the animals' urine.[8] If the body cannot properly synthesize collagen, health problems such as wrinkled skin, abnormal outgrowth of bone, arthritis, brittle bones, and arteriosclerosis may result.

Anecdotal evidence of fluoride's devastating effects have been documented in areas of Turkey and India where fluoride occurs naturally at levels as high as 5 ppm. For the residents of communities like Kizilcaoern, Turkey, brittle bones, stiff and painful joints, and weak muscle tone are almost the norm. As one German newspaper reported in a 1978 article on Kizilcaoern, "Forty-year-olds look like old men and women."[9]

In addition, Yiamouyiannis cites studies showing that fluoride may depress or inhibit the immune system by slowing the movement of white blood cells. This means that the cells cannot reach a foreign substance as quickly as may be needed to prevent the substance from circulating in the body.[10] Furthermore, fluoride interferes with thyroid activity. As little as 5 milligrams, the amount consumed daily by people drinking fluoridated water, has been shown to lower thyroid activity in humans.[11] Research published in the *Journal of Brain Research* in 1998 concluded that "the presence of fluoride in water may be linked with neurotoxic effects including changes to brain tissue not dissimilar to the changes found in Alzheimer's disease patients."[12] In September 1999 the *International Journal of Environmental Studies* published research which found that fluoridation increases lead absorption in children.[13]

Other research links fluoride to cancer, although no study indicates for certain that fluoride causes cancer. In 1991 the U.S. National Toxicology Program studied rats who consumed water with 100 or 175 ppm fluoride. Out of 362 rats, four developed unexpected bone cancer. The researchers declared that their study contained "equivocal evidence of carcinogenic activity." The study, however, raised concerns for people with osteoporosis who take fluoride supplements and live in highly fluoridated communities. When tested, these individuals have as much fluoride in their bones as the rats studied.[14]

In 1992 the State Board of Health in New Jersey found that "males aged 10–19 were nearly seven times more likely to get bone cancer if they lived in a fluoridated area than if they lived in a nonfluoridated municipality."[15] Also in the early 1990s, the National Cancer Institute reviewed cancer records from Iowa and Seattle between 1973 and 1987. They discovered a higher incidence of bone cancer among male children and teens in fluoridated areas.[16] The introduction of fluoride, however, did not coincide with the increase in cancer rates. Since no one knows the rate at which fluoride accumulates in the body, nor at what level it may interfere with bodily functions, the increase in cancer may never directly correspond to the introduction of fluoride, even if flouride does affect cancer.

Approximately 60 percent of U.S. communities fluoridate their water. The California Department of Health Services found that dental costs are higher in fluoridated areas. In July 1997 a group of EPA scientists "who assess the scientific data for Safe Drinking Water Act standards and other EPA regulations [went] on record against the practice of adding fluoride to public drinking water."[17] As an organization, however, the EPA remains in favor of fluoride.

The surprisingly long list of countries that prohibit fluoridation includes Austria, Belgium, China, Denmark, Finland, Germany, Holland, Hungary, Japan, the Netherlands, Norway, and Sweden. Only 10 percent of public drinking water in Britain is fluoridated.[18] Holland stopped fluoridation in 1976 and recommended fluoride supplements instead. In 1998, due to new evidence connecting fluoride with an increase in the incidence of cancer, arthritis, and neurological complaints, the country stopped recommending supplements.

John Colquhoun, a public health official in Auckland, New Zealand, spent considerable time standing on both sides of the issue. His story is one of an ardent fluoride proponent turned opponent. Colquhoun was a practicing dentist when the government appointed him as Principal Dental Officer, a position that oversees public water fluoridation. He advocated fluoridating all water in New Zealand and wrote articles for the *New Zealand Dental Journal* that promoted this agenda. He also chaired the country's Fluoridation Promotion Committee. In 1980 the government sent him on a world tour to promote fluoridation. He met with pro-fluoride scientists in America, Britain, and Europe, many of whom were conducting research on how fluoride affects large populations.

When he returned to New Zealand, he encountered a very surprising and unanticipated report. Recently gathered statistics of almost the entire child population of Auckland indicated that children in fluoridated areas had more fillings than did children in nonfluoridated areas. Studies from the rest of New Zealand showed similar trends. All in all, Colquhoun found enough evidence against fluoride to change his previously staunch opinion of how it should be used. He later became active in the International Society for Fluoride Research, established for "the purpose of advancement of research and dissemination of knowledge pertaining to the biological and other effects of fluoride on animal, plant, and human life."[19] The organization publishes the quarterly journal *Fluoride.*

We have always been exposed to fluoride. During the past fifty years we've been exposed to more fluoride than ever before. Our water, our toothpaste, and even our food contains fluoride. In spite of our safe threshold levels, fluoride sometimes mottles teeth. The most pressing unanswered question is: How does fluoride damage other parts of the body? As Colquhoun wrote in 1982, "Common sense should tell us that if a poison circulating in a child's body can damage tooth-forming cells, then other harm is likely."[20]

So where does this leave you and me, the consumers of dental care? I've never had a fluoride treatment, nor have my children. Based on my research, I find no reason for my children to take fluoride supplements. I can't help but wonder how many dentists have read the work of Yiamouyiannis for themselves. Are they aware of the most recent research on fluoride, which may not be published in ADA-sponsored medical journals? Do they know how other countries view the issue? Fortunately, researchers continue to investigate the safety of fluoridation. In the meantime, we must choose what we believe is healthiest for our children.

MERCURY AMALGAMS

The second hotly debated topic within the dental world concerns mercury amalgams, sometimes called silver fillings or mercury fillings. Growing up, I thought that silver fillings, as I always heard them referred to, were composed of silver. I didn't know that "amalgam" means an alloy containing mercury and at least one other metal. Dental amalgams are approximately 50 percent mercury, 30 percent silver, 13 percent tin, 2 percent copper, and a trace of zinc. When I had two cavities filled with amalgams back in 1981, I knew nothing about the controversy surrounding mercury fillings. I became aware of it when our homeopath suggested that my husband have his six amalgams replaced because studies had suggested that the mercury vapor and abraded particles that escape from fillings can cause a myriad of health problems. Only when I researched this chapter did I discover that pro-amalgamists and anti-amalgamists have been battling for 150 years.

The 150-Year War

Back in the 1800s, dentistry was not the regulated profession it is today. Basically, one could be a butcher, baker, or candlestick maker and still pull teeth on the side. Of course, there were professionals such as Dr. Chapin Harris, a medical doctor and dentist who authored textbooks on dentistry and helped found the first dental school. He was called a medical-dentist, while dentists like the neighborhood barber were called craftsmen-dentists.

In 1833, two profit-motivated Frenchmen by the last name of Crawcours came to America to introduce a product that had earned them a bundle of money in Europe: the dental amalgam. Until that point, medical-dentists filled cavities with gold. Since gold was expensive and time consuming to work with, dentistry was available only to a small segment of society. As the public soon discovered, via the Crawcourses' slick advertising, silver fillings were used at room temperature and went in painlessly. Besides, they were easy to shape once inside the tooth. Craftsmen-dentists quickly learned to work with amalgams. Because the fillings were affordable, dentistry became available to the masses. The Crawcours brothers hit it lucky again.

From the beginning, Dr. Chapin Harris criticized the use of amalgams. He knew, as did his peers, that mercury was extremely poisonous—more so, in fact, than arsenic or lead. Certainly, it was too toxic to insert into the mouth. In 1840 Chapin and other medical-dentists formed the American Society of Dental Surgeons (ASDS). The organization declared that the use of amalgams constituted malpractice. The craftsmen-dentists, who far outnumbered the medical-dentists, paid no heed and continued to profit from amalgams. In 1848 the ASDS disbanded due to low membership and lack of funds. Roughly a decade later, the amalgam dentists formed their own organization: the American Dental Association. The ADA has promoted the use of amalgams ever since.

The Current Debate

A 1995 ADA news release describes dental amalgams as a "safe, affordable, and durable material used to restore the teeth of more than 100 million Americans."[21] It also states that "dental amalgam has an indisputable safety record." The U.S. Public Health Service and the National Institutes of Dental Research agree that amalgam is safe and effective.

So why the ongoing debate? If the ADA has no qualms about using amalgam in teeth restoration, is it even worth our effort, as consumers, to question the safety of a material that has been used for over 150 years?

Anti-amalgamists have fired many flares of warning in an attempt to attract the attention of consumers, dentists, and public health officials. They believe that amalgams are a serious threat to a person's physical and emotional health. The culprit of the damage, they contend, is the mercury vapor and ions that escape from the amalgam and settle in the body. For many years, pro-amalgamists asserted that the mercury in fillings was inactive and therefore incapable of escaping from the teeth and disrupting health. In 1931, however, Dr. Alfred Stock showed that mercury vapor did indeed escape from fillings. His many articles on this subject were the target of much scorn, but new studies conducted in 1981 confirmed Dr. Stock's findings. In 1984 the ADA admitted for the first time that amalgam emits mercury vapor. At the same time, it added a clause to its code of ethics stating that dentists cannot ethically recommend that a patient have an amalgam removed unless they suspect a medical reason to do so. Today the ADA recognizes, as do all scientists, the extremely poisonous nature of elemental mercury, but the organization feels that no study has ever offered definitive proof that the minute amount of escaping mercury vapor causes harm to the body.

The question at the heart of the amalgam debate is not whether mercury vapor is toxic. As mentioned, mercury vapor is a known toxin. Instruments can measure the amount of mercury vapor and mercury ions in the mouth. Scientists know that chewing, particularly gum chewing, and drinking hot liquids accelerates the release of mercury vapor and ions. Rather, the question is whether a minuscule amount of mercury vapor emitted every day for years—even decades—can affect organs and systems in the human body. As with fluoride, no scientific study has determined absolutely, positively, without a doubt that mercury causes problems. Therefore, the ADA is unwilling to change its position that amalgams are safe and effective.

The anti-amalgamists claim that copious studies connect amalgam to serious health problems, including birth defects and multiple sclerosis. In pregnant women, for instance, the placental membrane prevents many substances from crossing into the fetus. Mercury vapor and methylmercury, a particularly poisonous form of mercury created by bacteria in the intestines, are fat soluble. Hence, they can cross the placental membrane, which is made up of fat molecules, and enter the fetus, where their effects are unknown. A study done in 1983 suggests that mercury may interfere with the transport of nutrients across the placenta into the fetus. "An inhibition of nutrient transport may cause fetal death, congenital malformations, or growth retardation," explains Sam Ziff and Dr. Michael Ziff in their book *Infertility & Birth Defects: Is Mercury from Silver Dental Fillings an Unsuspected Cause?*[22] Moreover, research since 1983 shows that mercury leaches into breast milk.[23]

These studies, among others, caused the Swedish Social Welfare and Health Administration to issue the following statement:

> As a first step in the process to eliminate the use of amalgam in dental fillings, comprehensive amalgam work on pregnant women shall be stopped in order to prevent mercury damage to the fetus.[24]

The German government has issued a similar warning against using amalgam in females of childbearing age.[25] The ADA has issued no such warning.

Anti-amalgamists also fear that mercury vapor affects the central nervous system. In 1983 Dr. Theodore Ingalls proposed in an article in the *American Journal of Forensic Medicine and Pathology* that the mercury escaping from root canals or dental amalgams could cause multiple sclerosis in middle age.[26] Other research links mercury to heart palpitations. Autopsies of Alzheimer's patients reveal high levels of mercury in brain tissue. Mercury also adversely affects the kidneys, which have difficulty filtering it out.[27] It can affect the thyroid and pituitary glands and can greatly affect emotions and mental stability, which has been known since the days of "mad hatters." Amalgams have been linked to "headaches, fatigue, mood swings, depression, suicidal thoughts, nervousness, fits of anger, shyness, and emotional outbursts."[28]

An estimated 50 tons of mercury is used every year in amalgams. Because the EPA classifies mercury as a hazardous waste, the ADA scrupulously instructs dentists on how to handle and dispose of amalgam. The mercury is yet another noxious substance for our Earth to try to absorb.

Should mercury amalgam remain innocent until proven guilty, or is there enough evidence to halt its use until we know for certain how it affects us physically and emotionally?

On a personal level, I find this issue easier to contend with than the fluoride or vaccine issues, mainly because no law mandates that cavities be filled with amalgam. I retain the freedom to choose a composite filling. If you're concerned about amalgams, all you have to do is find a dentist who is willing to use composites, a bis-gamma resin that is usually quartz filled and tooth colored. Composites are a bit more difficult to work with, which is one reason they cost more than amalgam. In the past, their longevity was questionable, but now they hold together for an estimated eight to ten years and sometimes longer. At any rate, what's more important, the life of the filling or the life of the patient?

If your child has an amalgam, you can have it removed and replaced with a composite. If one of my daughters needs a filling in the future, I certainly won't have it filled with amalgam, no matter how much I love my dentist. That's an easy choice. If she already had a mercury filling, I would choose to have it replaced because, for me, the issue is too unresolved. In 1990 my husband had his amalgams removed. He did not experience any overt change or improvement in his health. Although we'll never know if some subtle changes happened in his body, I find it reassuring to know that the potential for amalgams to harm his health is gone.

CARING FOR YOUR CHILD'S TEETH

So what's the best way to care for your child's teeth? Holistic and conventional dentistry agree on a number of points. First, dental care should begin at an early age. Second, don't put a baby to bed with a bottle of juice or milk. This could result in baby bottle syndrome, in which liquids pool against the teeth and cause decay.

When a child's teeth are new, wipe them gently with a cloth to clean them. When your child is around age two, start using the dry-brush method. Jostle the dry bristles of a soft brush on his teeth. Jostling breaks down plaque better than scrubbing. You may want to let the child hold the toothbrush and swish it around in his mouth. Don't worry if the bristles don't connect with the teeth. The idea is to get him accustomed to the feel of a brush in his mouth.

My children use nonfluoridated toothpaste. They weren't too interested in the hydrogen peroxide concoction, which doesn't have the most pleasant taste. If you prefer nonfluoridated toothpaste, you may have to go to a health food store, although some conventional grocers now carry Tom's of Maine toothpaste. Some of this brand's flavors are nonfluoridated.

You want your child to become familiar with the feel of clean teeth. Flossing increases that feeling. Until your child is coordinated enough to floss on her own, you will have to do it for her. Electric toothbrushes are another option, as is a water pick, which removes more food from between the teeth than does flossing.

Most important, feed your child nutritious foods. A healthful diet, combined with proper tooth care, fosters a healthy mouth.

CHAPTER 11

From Quacks to Qualified Professionals

Converse freely with quacks of every class and sex . . .
You cannot imagine how much a physician with a liberal mind may
profit from a few casual and secret visits to these people.

DR. BENJAMIN RUSH
(1756–1813)

It was one weird night.

Gregg and I drove through a chilly November rain at 9:00 P.M. en route to see a home video of a psychic surgery. A woman named Charlotte had said to meet her at a Marriott suite on the other side of town. An acquaintance of mine had put me in touch with Charlotte, who recently had been treated by a psychic healer in the Philippines and had videotaped her experience. Perhaps this was an option that could help Gregg; I must admit that the concept sounded a bit bizarre to both of us.

Two other couples were already seated in the hotel room when we arrived. Gregg, with his permanently curled fingers and thin hands, was the only person there with an obvious health problem. A plate of munchies beckoned from a small table, but my appetite had vanished somewhere along the freeway.

Charlotte got right down to business. About six months before, an MRI had shown a shadow of a growth near her pancreas, and her doctors had recommended exploratory surgery. Charlotte's mother had died of pancreatic cancer, and having witnessed her horrific experience with chemotherapy, Charlotte decided to try a radically different approach before committing to conventional care, even though her diagnosis was never definite.

Charlotte turned on the video. There she was, lying on a table, a man and a woman standing next to her. The man laid the tips of his index and middle fingers on Charlotte's torso and then pushed them through her skin. The woman sitting next to me inhaled sharply. The healer proceeded to pull out various pieces of long, whitish matter while his assistant dabbed at the small amount of blood trickling from the opening. I started to feel queasy and a little dizzy. I thought, I'm either going to pass out, leave the room, or get a grip. I decided to get a grip, and I managed to stay upright and focused. I hadn't expected to be so affected by a home video. After the healer pulled out quite a bit of whatever he was pulling out, he closed the wound by laying his fingertips over it. No stitches, no scar.

Charlotte said she had four one-hour sessions during her week's stay. She described the events in some detail. Upon returning home, she visited her physician, who ordered another MRI. Much to his amazement, the results were normal. Charlotte believed that during her trip she had healed. She then informed us that even though psychic surgery is not legal in the United States, we didn't need to travel to the Philippines: a healer was being smuggled into a nearby town to perform surgery. We could make an appointment with him if we wanted to do so.

Well, we never made the appointment, nor did we book a flight to the Philippines. I found some literature on psychic healing that explained how healers use energy and Spirit to perform their surgery. One publication included a litany of anecdotal success stories. Based on the video I saw and various conversations and readings, I believe that a healer can open the body with his hands. I felt no reason to doubt Charlotte's story or believe that she had anything but honest intentions. As for whether or not one truly can be healed through this type of therapy, for lack of personal experience I'll reserve judgment. For us, the option never felt quite right.

WHO'S THE QUACK?

Skeptics claim that psychic surgery is merely a magician's illusion. The person posing as a healer, explains Kurt Butler in his book *The Consumer's Guide to Alternative Medicine,* releases a bloodlike liquid from a capsule hidden in the cotton swabbing surrounding the supposed body opening. The healer-magician palms bits of animal tissue, which he appears to pull like a string of knotted scarves from the patient's torso. Any healing the patient experiences can be attributed to the placebo effect because the healer is nothing more than a quack.[1]

The dictionary defines *quack* as someone who pretends to possess medical skills or cure disease. A quack, in other words, is a con artist. The epitome of such a charlatan is the snake oil salesman of the 1800s, who promoted elixirs and potions purported to cure everything from a hangnail to debilitating arthritis. Yet in reality, the task of identifying a quack is a subjective endeavor. One's point of view ultimately determines who is the phony, the fraud, the con artist—the quack.

Throughout history, individuals who promoted the unconventional often have been labeled quacks. In the 1800s, Hungarian physician Ignaz Semmelweiss advised doctors and midwives to wash their hands in chloride of lime before touching a laboring or post-partum mother. Most doctors ignored Semmelweiss and never bothered to scrub between sessions with patients, despite the fact that doing so corresponded to a marked decrease in incidences of the often fatal childbed fever. A few decades later, the medical community similarly chided British surgeon Joseph Lister when he first recommended the antiseptic carbolic acid to clean surgical instruments, wounds, and dressings. Galileo, the man we now hail as a genius, was ostracized from many intellectual circles of his time. Eventually, he was condemned to house arrest for life because he championed the Copernican theory that the planets revolve around the sun. As he wrote to his friend and fellow astronomer, Johannes Kepler:

> What do you think of the foremost philosophers of this University? In spite of my oft-repeated efforts and invitations, it have refused, with the obstinacy of a glutted adder, to look at the planets or Moon or my telescope.[2]

In America during the 1800s, the American Medical Association (AMA) bristled at the "purveying of nostrums" and fought for legislation limiting the activities of individuals it deemed quacks. From the AMA's point of view, any person, doctor, or apothecary dealing in medicines outside of its protocol reeked of quackery. This included physicians and apothecaries who used herbal medicines and homeopathy. Some of the most influential homeopaths, like James Tyler Kent, were trained and licensed medical doctors, yet the AMA considered them quacks.

Today, the word *quack* remains a misused, dark term. Usually it means fraud, but sometimes the word is used synonymously with "incompetent." An incompetent medical professional, however, may not necessarily be a quack. Incompetency often arises from ignorance bred by a lack of knowledge or understanding. Incompetent professionals may not even be aware that they are incompetent. (Perhaps this makes them unconscious quacks.) On the other hand, some incompetents probably recognize their incompetency but, driven by a need to earn a living, practice their profession anyway.

As the demand for alternative medicine grows, the odds of encountering incompetency in the medical field increases due to the interplay of economic factors. In 1998 the median physician's income rose by 1 percent.[3] One way for doctors to boost income is to integrate alternative therapies into their practice. For you and me, the consumers of health care, this change has the potential to be a positive and a negative. The positive is that the supply of particular therapies, like herbal medicine and acupuncture, may keep closer pace with demand. The negative is that physicians or other practitioners may sell herbs or nutritional supplements simply to increase income, not because they believe the products actually work in the patient's best interest. The practitioners may not even be convinced of the healing effects of the alternative products they are selling.[4] Do such professionals fall under the category of con artist or incompetent?

Our task is difficult. We must try to discriminate between true visionaries and self-serving frauds, between legitimate unconventional practices and hocus-pocus quackery. Unfortunately, the lines of distinction blend like watercolors on wet canvas. Furthermore, the norm forever changes. Sometimes the unconventional remains far from the mainstream, as has psychic surgery, and sometimes it approaches the conventional, as has chiropractic. What constitutes quackery depends on one's perception; and, as always, perceptions vary. Thus, we are left with a Pandora's box of parameters defining quackery.

THE TWENTY-FIRST-CENTURY QUACKERY DEBATE

Rational Skeptics

On one side of the podium sit skeptics, represented by a myriad of organizations and publications. The Skeptics Society, for example, is a nonprofit group that publishes *Skeptic,* a magazine devoted to the "investigation of extraordinary claims and revolutionary ideas and the promotion of science and critical thinking."[5] The periodical defines skeptics as individuals who "must see compelling evidence" before they believe in something. Skeptics rely on reason, logic, and the scientific method developed in the sixteenth and seventeenth centuries to show that a theory can or cannot be temporarily accepted. Anecdotes and testimonials carry little weight in proving that systems like homeopathy or therapeutic touch actually work. For skeptics, the proof is in the randomized, placebo-controlled, double-blind clinical study, providing that the study has proper statistical analysis, long-term follow-up, and peer evaluation, and can be replicated by other scientists. Skeptics readily admit, however, that science is fallible and cannot prove everything.

One of the most vocal and widely published skeptics is Dr. Steven Barrett, a retired psychiatrist and consumer advocate for health fraud. His extensive Web site, www.quackwatch.com, reviews over thirty alternative therapies under the subheading "Questionable Products, Services, and Theories." Here, acupuncture and chiropractic become highly questionable therapies. Naturopaths are not trustworthy, and homeopathy is the "ultimate fake." In fact, Barrett writes that the FDA should not allow the "worthless products" of homeopathy to be marketed with claims that they are effective. In 1994, forty-two prominent critics who call alternative therapies like homeopathy "quackery" and "pseudosciences" petitioned the FDA to curb the sale of homeopathic products, citing the fact that the products are not regulated as over-the-counter drugs and, therefore, are not subject to the same safety tests.

If homeopathic remedies were in fact subject to the same safety tests as conventional drugs, homeopathy could easily be eliminated from the marketplace, since the sciences used to test pharmaceutical drugs—such as organic chemistry—have difficulty proving the efficacy of homeopathic medicines. In order to be effective, homeopathic remedies must be matched to the patient's symptoms; a double-blind placebo study would need to be modified to include this stipulation before it could be considered accurate. Finally, the remedies are best explained by the energy theories found in certain branches of quantum physics, theories which are still considered unconventional by mainstream medical standards.

The National Council Against Health Fraud (NCAHF), a private organization started by Dr. William Jarvis, another well-published skeptic, also advises consumers against alternative practices. In regard to homeopathy, the NCAHF recommends that no one use homeopathic products or consult with homeopaths. Furthermore, "basic scientists are urged to be proactive in opposing the marketing of homeopathic remedies because of conflicts with known physical laws."[6] The NCAHF encourages states to abolish homeopathic licensing boards.

Dr. Wallace Sampson is a clinical professor at Stanford University School of Medicine and edits the *Scientific Review of Alternative Medicine,* sponsored by the Council for Scientific Medicine. This organization also leans toward rational skepticism, although Sampson claims that "it will reject no claim because it fits, or fails to fit, some paradigm." Even so, can we scientifically test a theory from one paradigm using a theory from another paradigm?

Other Skeptics

On the other side of the quackery debate are citizens, scientists, and medical professionals who prudently accept alternative medicines. This group excludes those individuals who blindly try every therapy, every fad diet, and every herb they hear or read about. Rather, here sit individuals like Dr. Andrew Weil, who describes himself as an open-minded skeptic. Although both rational skeptics and open-minded skeptics rely on rational thinking and logic, an important difference divides the two groups. Unlike rational skeptics, open-minded skeptics are willing to test the waters without demanding that quantitative science justify every therapy. If a therapy has been used successfully for an extensive period of time—say three thousand years, as in the case of Ayurveda and TCM—then it may be worth integrating into medicine even if basic science cannot crack its codes of success. Moreover, personal experience and anecdotal and clinical evidence are taken into account by open-minded skeptics when determining if a therapy is safe and effective.

Would public demand for alternative medicine be so high if personal experience did not affirm that therapies like chiropractic, massage, acupuncture, oriental medicine, and herbs help heal illness? I'm not sure that I would have accepted much of alternative medicine without personal experience. My very first experience with any alternative occurred in 1985 when my back muscles locked in place. The emergency room physician prescribed a few muscle relaxants. After three days of being lost in a drug-induced haze with still minimal mobility, I concluded that my back was not healing well. I decided to consult a chiropractor. I had never been to one before. After the first treatment, I could get out of bed by myself and move around slowly. By the third manipulation, the pain had subsided significantly. What's more, I was mobile and back at work. I have since visited chiropractors many times for back troubles. Rational skeptics roll their eyes at this kind of anecdotal evidence.

About a year after my first chiropractic experience, I felt a lump at the base of my throat every time I swallowed. An ear, nose, and throat specialist examined me and said I was experiencing acid reflux, in which the acids from the stomach creep up the esophagus and settle in the throat. Take these pills, he directed. "These pills" were great! After a week of hovering an inch or so above reality, I felt that perhaps this was more than a physical issue. When the problem started, I had been unusually stressed. I made another appointment, this time at a wellness clinic with a therapist who taught me how to use visualization and breathing techniques to reduce stress. I promptly stopped the medication. Two weeks into using these new skills, the lump disappeared. For years now, visualization and imagery techniques, along with diaphragmatic breathing, have eased me through many stressful situations, including the challenges of natural childbirth.

One of the best testimonials for an alternative therapy I have heard comes from a friend who had an acute rash, terribly itchy and unattractive, on her neck. She refused to use a steroid cream to clear it up. Instead, she went to an acupuncturist. When she told me this, I thought she had picked the wrong alternative modality. I guess I thought acupuncture was more for pain than anything else. Sarah said that after only two treatments the rash cleared up and never returned. Placebo? Coincidence? Sound and effective treatment? Your view of science, medicine, and healing will determine your answer.

One organization that is very interested in the subjective experience of healing is the Institute of Noetic Sciences (IONS) located in Sausalito, California. *Noetic* is the Greek word for "intuitive knowing." A noetic science takes into account the world of inner experience. It considers consciousness in all aspects of science and medicine. Much of IONS's work strives for a deeper understanding of our spiritual nature and attempts to determine why some people heal while others don't. One IONS-sponsored research project evaluated metastatic cancer patients who had survived their illness for twenty or more years. Researchers were interested in the emotional and mental factors, such as the individuals' perception of disease, that may have helped these patients survive. The study found that these cancer patients did not regard their disease or recovery as unusual. Another study now underway is focusing on how a specific meditation affects immune functions. Another is addressing the issue of whether individuals can use their minds to influence the material world. Is the mind capable of altering organic substances? Can it really heal the body?

ENERGY MEDICINE: OUR NEWEST FRONTIER OR OUR LATEST QUACKERY?

Some open-minded skeptics also embrace the concept of energy. For the most part, rational skeptics find the idea about as solidly grounded as packing peanuts in a hurricane, but I would be remiss if I didn't include a discussion of energy. You see, I knew when I started to write this book that somewhere I would have to incorporate concepts of energy, but I wasn't quite sure how to do this. In fact, the mere notion of mentioning energy, chi, prana, and vital energy—which are basically all the same thing—made me squirm. It all sounds so weird, so far out, so mystical. We can relate to the discoveries of new genes and drugs and even get excited about them, but when someone mentions vital energy we shake our heads in disbelief. So I planned to tuck the energy stuff here and there and not make a big deal about it. Ha! Was I wrong. When I started writing, energy concepts surfaced naturally and almost immediately. After all, how can one talk about Ayurveda, homeopathy, TCM, and herbal medicine without focusing on energy, the very concept upon which these systems are all based?

More and more scientific studies are focusing on energy. At the University of Arizona, Dr. Gary Schwartz—director of the Human Energy Systems Lab; professor in the departments of psychology, medicine, neurology, and psychiatry; and coauthor of *The Living Energy Universe*—researches mind-body medicine, energy medicine, and spiritual medicine. Using an EEG amplifier in one study, Dr. Schwartz quantified electromagnetic fields created by physical movements of the human body. In another study, individuals open to receiving communication from others located at a distance were able to detect when communication had been sent. Such research eventually may validate energy medicine.

QUACKBUSTING QUESTIONS AND PATIENT GUIDELINES

So who's the quack and who's the quackbuster? Are an ounce of experience, a gram of belief, and a beaker full of scientific studies sufficient to identify the quackery suspect in the lineup of alternative therapies? Without a doubt, quacks and quack therapies stealthily amble around health food stores, the Internet, and even doctors' offices. Unfortunately, there is no foolproof way to detect them. The best that conscientious consumers can do is ask some quackbusting questions and follow some patient guidelines.

Questions

Is the supplement, procedure, therapy, or remedy touted as a miracle worker?

Nothing cures everything! Don't buy it or do it if it claims to eliminate all health problems.

Is the practitioner licensed?

This isn't a bad question to ask, but in some ways it's rather superficial. Licensing requirements vary greatly from state to state and from profession to profession. To practice acupuncture legally in Arizona, for instance, all practitioners—including M.D.s—need to graduate from or complete training in a program approved by the state's Acupuncture Board of Examiners. The program must have a minimum of 1,850 hours, including 800 hours of clinical experience. In at least twenty-seven other states, M.D.s are allowed to practice acupuncture without any specialized training. Scary, huh? In some of these states, other professionals—like dentists, chiropractors, or those offering only acupuncture—can become licensed if they complete required educational courses and have clinical experience.[7]

Perhaps a better way to choose a practitioner is to inquire about the person's background. In other words, what is the practitioner's perspective of health and healing? Is her training purely allopathic, in which case she views disease in only one way, or does she have training in, or an understanding of, classical medicines like TCM, which incorporate a more holistic view of the body? As a patient, you need—and have the right—to ask these questions.

Is the practitioner recommending supplements or therapies for the remainder of your life or your child's life?

Supplements, when used judiciously, can help correct imbalances in the body. However, this does not mean that, once started, they must be continued for life. If the symptoms disappear or change, talk to your practitioner about altering the dosage or discontinuing the supplement. Be particularly careful of giving children, whose bodies are still developing, supplements for long periods of time.

What kind of relationship do you have with your practitioner(s)?

When I consult a practitioner, I expect to work with him at eye level even though he may be more knowledgeable about medicine. A condescending or disparaging attitude is uncalled for by either doctor or patient. Nor can I work with anyone who openly condemns my choices. My daughters' first pediatrician firmly believed in vaccines, yet when I told him that I did not want to vaccinate the girls, he accepted my decision. He offered his point of view, but he never made me feel like a neglectful mother or an incompetent human being. He respected my decision.

GUIDELINES

Question and learn

Health care practitioners are in a marvelous position to teach and patients are in a prime position to learn. Yet each must be willing to do so. As a patient, ask as many questions as possible. Don't let fear keep you immobile. Become as educated as possible. This may require time and extra effort. Reading a pamphlet on the pros and cons of vaccines ten minutes before your child gets a round of shots is not adequate education. You need to gather as much information as possible and digest it before making all-important health decisions.

Listen to and trust your intuition

We're taught to rely on professionals and on science, but our intuition—that feeling that something is either not quite right or, conversely, just what we need—can be incredibly wise. If a therapy, treatment, or recommendation doesn't feel right, try to discern why. One neurologist recommended that my husband try experimental chemotherapy. Gregg's intuition said, "No go." Doctors have followed "hunches" for centuries. Patients can do the same.

Baby Brittany

I ran into Carol while dropping the girls off at gymnastics. A few seasons back, our husbands had coached our kids' soccer team together. We started chatting. The conversation meandered to children and stuffy spring noses and other health issues, and soon we discovered that we had both had experiences with holistic medicine. While the girls tumbled around indoors, Carol related her saga.

She and her husband, Mike, had adopted baby Brittany when she was four days old. During her first year of life, Brittany came down with a fever that lasted about three days, followed by a distinctive red rash. "All is normal," the doctor assured Carol and Mike, "it's roseola infantum." As with chicken pox, once a child has roseola, she won't get it again. Brittany, however, defied the odds. Over the next nine months, the fever and rash returned three more times. "Highly unusual," the doctor muttered.

The next year, Brittany's fevers, sans rash, started after the family's big Thanksgiving reunion and recurred every other month lasting about four days until June and the start of warmer weather. Although her tonsils always swelled, tests for strep came back negative. For each fever, the doctor recommended rest and acetaminophen.

The following fall, when Brittany was two years old, a new fever pattern started. Now she contended with weeklong fevers every month. Carol brought her weakened daughter to the pediatrician for almost every fever, but no other symptoms appeared besides swollen tonsils. The doctor again prescribed acetaminophen as needed. In the spring, the fevers began occurring every few weeks. The doctor suggested alternating ibuprofen with the acetaminophen. Again, Carol diligently followed his suggestions. He had been a colleague of her father's, a general practitioner, and Carol's pediatrician. Naturally, Carol felt weighted with worry, but she felt no reason not to trust the physician. Again, the fevers ended in June.

They returned at Thanksgiving. Brittany, now three years old, had roughly three days of health between fevers that lasted from one to two weeks. For one three-week stretch, her temperature hovered around 102 degrees, sometimes creeping as high as 106 degrees. Carol and Mike frantically watched their daughter grow more and more lethargic. Listless, Brittany spent each day on the couch. Her white blood cell count remained normal. Her tonsils were swollen, but her ears looked clear and she never developed strep. The doctor referred Brittany to an ear, nose, and throat specialist, who recommended adenoid surgery and ear tubes to help any resulting drainage.

After the surgery, Brittany started vomiting on a regular basis and quickly lost weight. She was like a newborn, unable to play or walk around. Carol left the house with her as little as possible. She and Mike had never bothered to have Brittany baptized, but now, uncertain how much longer their frail daughter would be able to cling to life, they proceeded with the ceremony.

Carol became desperate. As a last resort, she decided to follow a friend's recommendation and see a Chinese doctor. You don't need an appointment, the friend instructed. Just show up at the shop.

Carol was a bundle of nerves as she stepped from the chilly spring air into the Chinese herbal store with Brittany in her arms. Jars of herbs lined three of the walls and were stacked almost floor to ceiling. A woman behind the counter told Carol to take a seat in one of the chairs set in the middle of the store where four other people also waited. Within thirty minutes, Carol was ushered into a tiny back room probably no bigger than 8 by 8 feet.

A large bookcase rested against the wall opposite the door. There was just enough room between it and the desk for the doctor to sit. His granddaughter sat in a nearby chair. As Carol related the events of the past four years, the granddaughter translated Carol's words into Chinese. The doctor had Carol lay Brittany across his desk. He waggled his tongue at Brittany in an attempt to get her to waggle hers back so he could examine it. The doctor became very disgruntled when he heard about the treatments Brittany had undergone. "His nostrils flared," said Carol.

The granddaughter translated as the doctor explained Brittany's condition. Her immune system was almost nonexistent. Her past treatments had contributed to her decline by impeding the healing process. The doctor prescribed some Chinese herbs. "Fever not come again," said the granddaughter. "And she grow big. Not so skinny anymore." She held her hand above the desk, indicating how tall Brittany would grow. Carol started to cry with relief. Might this work? she wondered.

The doctor prescribed one week's worth of herbs. Carol was told to return on the seventh day for another batch. The fifteen-minute appointment and medicine cost a total of thirty dollars.

As instructed, Carol boiled the herbs into a thick, dark, nasty-tasting tea. She persuaded Brittany to drink it in a little shot glass. "Okay, down it goes," Carol would say. Brittany would do a shot of tea, then follow with an apple juice chaser. After two days, Brittany's fever disappeared. Carol and Mike braced themselves for its return, but it didn't come back on schedule.

At the end of the week, Carol and Brittany returned to the Chinese doctor. After a ten-minute exam, he prescribed another week of herbal tea. By the end of the second week, Brittany no longer spent the entire day on the couch. The doctor visits and herbal tea treatments continued for two more weeks. By the end of the fourth

week, much to Carol and Mike's delight, Brittany had to be repri-
manded for needling her older brother. The cost of all the treatments
totaled $180.

The doctor told Carol to bring Brittany back once a month for
a year to make sure that her immune system remained strong. At
each visit, he recommended some mild-tasting herbal medicine that
looked like cough drops. Listening to Carol's story, I watched eight-
year-old Brittany skip rope on the sidewalk near where Carol and I
sat. Her last consultation had been three years ago.

Placebo? Quackery? Coincidence? Legitimate medicine?

Carol and Mike call it a miracle.

CHAPTER 12

The Spirit Within

The true self within each of us is our spiritual being. This true self is a spark of divinity that seeks to emerge into consciousness, for such an emergence is the next step in the evolution of our species.

DAVID MARSHAK
THE COMMON VISION: PARENTING AND EDUCATING FOR WHOLENESS

Like most three-year-olds, C.J. loved to dress up. The other kids at preschool knew that the sparkly blue skirt belonged to C.J. Every day during free time, C.J. hoisted the flouncy frock to waist level. At home, C.J. insisted on wearing "hair"—a dishtowel wrapped around the head and knotted with a band at the neck. When a towel wasn't donned, various barrettes dangled from C.J.'s hair. C.J. loved Pocahontas, with her long black braids. Mesmerized by music and dance, particularly Irish dance, C.J. spent much time on tiptoes. C.J. pursued what made C.J. feel good.

C.J.'s parents wisely did not interfere with their child's preferences, even though C.J. does not stand for Christina Jane or Clarissa Jo. It stands for Christopher John. At the age of three, this child was not cognizant of the parameters of sexuality that society imposes on children, even very young children. C.J. simply followed his spirit's deepest desires, and his parents granted him the freedom to do so.

What if C.J.'s mom and dad disapproved of his "hair"? What if they forbade him to wear plastic red and pink barrettes? What if the preschool teacher allowed him to claim the blue skirt only once a week? Most likely, C.J. would hurt on some level. Potentially, his physical, emotional, and spiritual bodies would suffer the pangs of limited make-believe. Perhaps, at the very least, his spirit would be bruised. As with any injury, it would require time and the proper care to heal.

Spirit is an integral part of human health. When it comes to health, however, we are inclined to focus on physical symptoms—and maybe on mental and emotional symptoms—but we often disregard our spiritual well-being. As with any other part of us, our spirit needs nurturing. Spirit is the deepest, most conscious part of our being. We are born with a completely developed spirit, and like a delicate seedling in a spring garden, our spirits must be properly cared for and fed as we mature from infants into adults. Through spiritual nourishment, our consciousness evolves, bringing us clarity and awareness and imparting a richer meaning to our human experience.

Spirit is a key component of classical systems of medicine including Ayurveda and TCM. In these holistic philosophies, spirituality and health are inseparable; the focus is on healing the entire person, which includes the person's spirit. One foundation of all classical medicines is to return a person, through some kind of teaching, therapy, and proper diet, to a natural state of being. If we stray from this natural state, we jeopardize our health. Disease may start. In his book *Care of the Soul*, Thomas Moore writes, "If the link between life experience and deep imagination is inadequate, then we are left with a division between life and soul, and such a division will always manifest itself in symptoms."[1] Hence, we must become aware of all that is natural to humans and to the environment that sustains humans. Is it natural, for instance, to add chemicals to food, to the environment, or to our bodies? Is it natural to vaccinate?

Classical medicines encourage us to learn about and practice spirituality, just as they encourage us to pursue a healthful diet. The care of the soul, or spirit, begins in childhood. As a child grows, her parents must identify the sustenance best suited to that child's spiritual needs. A spiritual fingerprint is as unique as a physical fingerprint. In other words, what satiates your child's spiritual hunger may differ from your own needs as much as Aretha Franklin differs from Pavarotti. Through wisdom, patience, and an understanding of the nature of spirit, we can all learn to feed children their optimum spiritual diet.

SPIRIT AND CREATIVITY

The French writer Emile Zola said, "I am an artist. I am here to live out loud." Regardless of our vocation, education, or cultural background, we all qualify as artists. Our spirit is like a bottomless jar of creativity that we continuously spread across the tapestry of life. In fact, every single human being enters this life clutching a piece of the great tapestry. From birth on, we draw, paint, dance, write, weave, and sing onto this marvelous creation. We dab paint onto it when we pour our morning cereal. We waltz across its surface as we choose the color and texture of our clothes for the day. When we drive to work, clean the kitchen counters, return phone calls, listen to music, or sit absorbed in silence, we sing melodies onto it. Consciously or unconsciously, we weave every action, thought, feeling, and prayer onto this living, pulsating tapestry.

We constantly create. The creative spirit penetrates our every dimension. The metabolism of our physical bodies reflects this creativity as it replaces old cells with new cells. Every seven days or so, the body completely "re-creates" itself. Without this creativity, we would disintegrate into formless blobs of withered cells, less organized than amoebas bumping against each other.

Children are bright, bold reflections of the creative spirit. As Wordsworth wrote, they come "trailing clouds of glory." For the most part, they have not yet acquired the practical, learned responses of the psyche. Within our daily web of chores, work, and child rearing, one of our greatest responsibilities is to recognize children as creative beings. It's so easy to get caught up in the energy of our own creating that we forget to look directly at our children's creative processes and allow them sufficient room to flourish.

I discovered this one night during the bedtime bath routine. The upstairs was so messy that it had become a disaster area, and I had reached my breaking point. As two-year-old Hannah played with her toys in the tub and Gregg read on a stool nearby, I attempted to create order out of chaos. I went from room to room, depositing clean laundry in dresser drawers and closets and picking up errant toys strewn in my path. When I finished my chores, I proceeded to the bathroom, which Gregg was just leaving. I forgot, however, to step out of my creating and give space to Hannah's. I burst through the bathroom door into a now warm, moist grotto where a toddler meditated in watery silence. I completely shattered her creation. Hannah, startled, started to cry. I realized belatedly what I had destroyed.

In order to tread respectfully around a child's creation, we must take time to recognize the motions of creativity. This is usually not difficult, because the creative spirit manifests a particular focus. A child absorbed in creative play exudes discipline, meaning, and direction. The atmosphere resonates with his contentment and settled energy. By exploring the physical environment with all of his senses, the child, through creating, experiments with life. We might say that the creative spirit images life; it presents itself through the child's "image-ination."

Take note of how your child expresses himself. What emotions, actions, sounds, colors, and textures does he incorporate into creations?

The next step is not to interfere. Provided that the child's choices are not harmful, we must harness the urge to promote our adult preferences, lest we destroy the child's creation like seawater surging over a delicate sand castle. In my opinion, my daughters look adorable in pink—hot pink, pale pink—all shades of pink complement their blond hair. I have learned, however, not to purchase pink clothes. They never leave the dresser drawer. For whatever reason, pink does not resonate with their creative expression; it resonates with mine.

Your child's environment is important to observe. Can your child create freely in the environments where she spends time? Environment includes not only physical surroundings, but also the intangible atmosphere that sparks sensations and feelings that, in turn, indelibly press upon the mind, body, and spirit. Parents and educators assume much of the responsibility of providing space that encourages children to freely create but that also has boundaries— preferably smooth, rounded boundaries that are unlikely to puncture the spirit. Politeness, respect, safety, and consideration stroke the spirit like a piece of soft cotton; intimidation, disrespect, and excessive control irritate the human spirit like scratchy wool against tender skin.

Elle spent one enjoyable school year at her preschool, but during the summer her attitude seemed to shift. She had just turned four. The looser summer schedule incorporated sprinkler time and more art time, activities that normally piqued her interest. By midsummer, however, she complained each morning about having to go to school. I worked out of our home, and her half days at preschool afforded me uninterrupted desk time, so I was reluctant to change the routine. In addition, I recently had become more active in the school community and was enjoying meeting new people and immersing myself in new projects. Besides, Hannah enjoyed the setting and never complained. I patted Elle's hand and kept reassuring her that she would have a good time with her friends and then could come home and swim and ride her bike.

She survived the summer and in the fall started the school year with a new teacher. Her new schedule seemed problem free. But, one day in September, when I picked her up, Elle burst into tears for no apparent reason. I decided to spend some time with her in class, a custom not routinely followed by parents at that particular school. I soon saw the problem. The school, which was run by experienced, loving teachers, had too many children, too many classes, and too much hubbub for Elle. She had always been shy. Now, I saw that her shyness had grown rather than abated. The day I helped in class, Elle stiffened when another child asked to join in her play, and she was unresponsive when the teachers gave attention to her. I finally recognized her unhappiness.

Other children, including Elle's sister, Hannah, thrived at that school, but Elle needed a different environment. I felt that a smaller school offering a totally different experience would awaken her subdued spirit. I investigated five or six schools. The one Gregg and I eventually chose was much smaller and offered a unique philosophy about educating children. After a month at the new school, she started blossoming and then bloomed into a happy, outgoing child. This school's environment matched her spirit better.

Spirit and Experience

Experience begins in the womb. Studies show that a fetus can identify its mother's voice among other sounds. Once a baby is born, every experience, be it a burnt tongue or hurt feeling, a loving hug or gentle praise, imprints itself on that child's sensitive spirit. Experiences mold the spirit, pushing here and there, sometimes lightly, sometimes firmly. At the same time, the spirit forms experience. What we call an adventurous spirit, for example, will lead one to different experiences than will a timid spirit. Thus, experience and spirit are intertwined; experience shapes spirit and spirit shapes experience. One way we can help our children's spirits grow healthy is to influence their experiences positively.

Helping children have positive experiences does not necessitate removing all obstacles from their path. One morning while visiting a friend, I watched three children mill around the toy bin. The youngest, Ryan, started pulling on a toy with a long handle. The handle connected to a plastic bubble encasing colored balls that bounced around noisily when the toy was pushed. The bubble was buried below other toys, and Ryan was trying his fifteen-month-old hardest to extract it. I was inclined to jump up and help him out, but his mother was sitting near me and I thought it best to leave that action to her. I noticed that she was keeping an eye on him. He worked at the toy for a good ten minutes, manipulating it in circles and tugging at it, until finally he pulled it triumphantly from the bin. The toy caught the eye of another toddler who grabbed it out of Ryan's hands. "Erin," said Ryan's mother immediately, "please give that back to Ryan. He worked very hard to get it out."

Children also learn by imitating. They observe the actions of adults and then mimic those actions. Through imitation, they experience their environment and, in the process, learn. "Can I help?" is a preschooler's common refrain to a parent who is folding laundry or cooking. I remember my mother letting me wash the windows when I was three or four years old. Although I probably thoroughly smeared them, what I remember is the feel of the cool, damp cloth gliding over the glass, the pungent smell of ammonia, and the overall satisfaction that I could work alongside and help Mama.

I was fascinated by fourteen-month-old Hannah the day I took the extralong route home from the grocery store, hoping that she might snooze in her car seat. No such luck. I continued to hear indecipherable chattering. When I glanced in the rearview mirror, I saw her kissing her doll's feet one at a time and cooing to it. I realized that she was copying my actions; when I changed her diapers, I always smooched the balls of her feet. Of course, she then uttered some stern gibberish at the doll, which made me reflect on how I spoke to her at other times.

Spirit and Education

As we've discussed, children learn through creative and experiential processes. These processes are integral to education, whether the learning occurs at school or within a peer group. While we can't always influence creativity and experience in peer groups, we certainly can control it in curriculums and classrooms. But how much space does education allocate to creativity? What type of experiences do educational systems give our children?

Most of us want schools to teach our children. We hope that our children will eventually graduate from high school with strong reading, writing, and math skills. Some states now require seniors to pass a test proving that they have adequate knowledge in these areas. The test serves as a checks-and-balances system for curriculums, teachers, and students. Low test scores may point to omissions in the curriculum. These standardized tests reflect an educational system that focuses on memory and reasoning skills. Creativity and experience are relegated to the back burner; they are not needed to graduate. They are needed, however, to develop consciousness and to experience a full life.

We focus so intently on children's grades and standardized test scores that we seem to forget that learning stems from an inborn curiosity about life. As Richard Lewis reminds us in his book *Living by Wonder: The Imaginative Life of Childhood,*

> How stifling it is for many children in our schools to find after kindergarten (in some cases before) that the prerequisites of getting ahead in school are to divide play from work, imagination from fact, feeling from truth. How confusing it must be for children to be told that their senses (hence their bodies) are not where they learn, and that real learning takes place only in the citadels of their intellect.[2]

Through the experience of playing, imaging, and creating, we acquire wisdom. We breathe in experience. The Latin word for "breath" is the root word for "inspire." You might say that we learn through "inspire-ation." The practices of yoga, tai chi, and meditation all use breathing to connect the body and mind to the spirit. Can we logically connect spirit to learning? Would recognizing spirit in the educational process make that process more fulfilling, more expansive, more nurturing of the whole child? After all, we did not acquire the wisdom that helps us as parents and adults by memorizing compartmentalized facts.

My experience with holistic education came from a Waldorf school. When Elle switched preschools, she started in a Waldorf system, which, at the time, I was not very familiar with. After a bit of reading and talking with Waldorf parents, my deductive reasoning and intuition told me that it would be an appropriate place for Elle. Our Waldorf experience mirrored that of my journey from conventional to alternative medicine. To put it succinctly, it changed my paradigm of what education should be.

The Waldorf system was the innovation of Rudolf Steiner, who opened the first Waldorf school in 1919 in Stuttgart, Germany. You may recall from the nutrition chapter that Steiner also created bio-dynamic farming. A brilliant philosopher and scientist, he formulated a holistic philosophy of living called anthroposophy, which focuses on the lifelong development of body, mind, and spirit. Steiner extended this philosophy to medicine, as well as education. Today, anthroposophic doctors in the United States and many other countries practice Steiner's holistic medicine.

A Waldorf education focuses on the head, heart, and hands, which represent the triune of spirit, emotions, and body. The ultimate aim of a Waldorf education is to foster a lifelong love of learning and instill a reverence for the world's wonder and beauty. Steiner proposed that when this occurs, children grow into balanced and creative human beings who use their imaginations to the fullest potential.

From birth through about age seven, children learn through imitation and movement. In a Waldorf kindergarten, children spend considerable time at imaginative play using toys made of natural materials like wood or wool. This encourages a relationship with nature. Storytelling is also prominent in the curriculum. Fairy tales are told—not read—to children and are often enacted with puppets. Letters and numbers and other intellectual endeavors are not introduced until the grades.

From ages seven through puberty, children learn through imagination and artistic expression. In grade school, writing, drawing, and storytelling are central to all lessons, including mathematics. Work sheets and printed textbooks are not found in Waldorf schools. Children create their own textbooks, which are literally works of art. From first to eighth grades, they also learn to play instruments, including the recorder and stringed instruments; speak two foreign languages; knit and sew; and do woodworking. In addition, eurythmy, a type of physical movement that incorporates music and speech, is part of each school day.

From puberty on, learning occurs through intellectual thought and abstract reasoning. In Waldorf high schools, students approach the arts and humanities from an intellectual perspective, although creativity, imagination, and physical movement continue to play important roles in the educational process. Students participate in orchestra, sing in choir, and pursue weaving and other art forms. Although quite different from public education, a Waldorf education prepares students well for higher learning.

During all stages of childhood and in all grades, the Waldorf system strongly discourages TV viewing. Because TV and videos provide words and images, the brain does not receive the stimulus that it requires to respond with creative inner imaging. Television fails to develop the imagination. For children to learn, says Dr. Jane Healy in her essay "Understanding TV's Effects on the Developing Brain," they must "personally investigate the three-dimensional world."[3]

What can kids investigate when they are under the hypnotic influence of television? Normally, children are kinetic bundles of energy. Sit them in front of the boob tube, though, and they transform into glassy-eyed lumps. In his book *The Treatment of Children by Acupuncture*, Dr. Julian Scott writes:

> The overstimulation provided by television causes tension to build up in the body. In the normal way this would be relieved in children by running around and other outdoor activities, but with television the children remain nearly motionless, allowing the tension to transform to heat.[4]

Too much heat unbalances the body and can lead to illness or exacerbate illness.

Television also affects behavior. According to the American Academy of Pediatrics, children who watch a lot of television are more likely to act aggressively and tend to be less empathetic. In addition, television frightens with monsters and scary plots, as well as with real violence. Certainly, it confuses young children who cannot differentiate between programs and commercials.[5]

Despite such drawbacks, children spend hours in front of the television screen. The average preschooler watches 27 hours of TV each week, which breaks down to about 3.5 hours a day. By the time this preschooler graduates from high school, he will have racked up 20,000 hours in front of the television versus 11,000 hours in the classroom.[6] To remind us that there are alternatives to television, the organization TV-Turnoff Network instituted a National TV-Turnoff Week, which encourages television addicts to "turn off the television and turn on the creativity."

If you feel that your children watch too much television, try limiting their viewing time. Take note of what other experiences they create instead. You may be surprised. When we limited TV time, the kids and their friends were forced to play. Now they spend a lot of time playing house and building forts, as well as doing art projects and making a general mess of things—but that's okay. I can see the imagination and creative processes in full swing.

Perhaps the idea of a holistic education that incorporates spirit, emphasizes creativity and imagination in all subjects, and discourages television and other addictive media will gather steam. For now, children sometimes spend more time coloring between the lines on work sheets than creating their own pictures.

Cathy's son James loved art. One day his kindergarten class painted frogs on white paper that were then pasted onto a background of green construction paper. The masterpieces were hung on a wall outside the classroom for students and parents to admire. When Cathy saw the paintings, she couldn't help but wonder why they were all green. Why not let them paint pink frogs or purple polka-dotted frogs or rainbow frogs? The teacher said that she didn't want the children to grow up thinking that frogs were not green. Reality hits soon enough, Cathy countered. If all the frogs are green, continued Cathy, the kids will be inclined to make judgments about who paints a more realistic—and, therefore, better—frog. Why not let them delight in a variety of frogs? Her comments fell on deaf ears.

Too bad Cathy couldn't consult Picasso. He would have concurred that not all frogs are green.

Spirit Food

We can dish a variety of spiritual food onto our children's platters. Fairy tales, rock collecting, dress-up, jokes, prayers, belly laughs, hugs—the spiritual morsels are many. What's more, they cost far less than organic foods but are just as important, if not more so, for big and little bodies. Moreover, they are easy to prepare. I only have to remind myself not to let my preoccupations prevent me from sharing and tasting these treats with my children.

Laughter

My friend Jane and I joined the kids, aged nine months to six years, at the table for lunch.

"All right, who's got a joke?" asked Jane.

Now this was something I never did with my kids. I slouched in my chair, hoping one of the less inhibited would speak up. I stutter through jokes, forget parts, and more than once have faked a laugh when I didn't get the punch line. I am basically joke challenged.

Much to my relief, Jane's six-year-old son David volunteered.

"Knock-knock."

"Who's there?" the other kids chimed in.

"Waddle."

"Waddle who?"

"Waddle you buy me for my birthday?" David said, eyes sparkling.

Grins and giggles erupted around the table.

Tommy, a three-year-old, started another joke. It was so convoluted and long and nonsensical that it sent Jane and me into spasms of laughter.

Jokes started flying fast and furious. Peals of pure mirth reverberated around the room. The baby banged his high chair tray, no one ate, but everyone's stomach muscles felt tight from laughing. We were getting a laughter workout.

Laughter is infectious. It is also healing. Just refer to Dr. Norman Cousins, who describes in his book *Anatomy of an Illness* how, by watching funny movies, he laughed his way from a serious condition, in which his body stopped properly synthesizing collagen, back to good health. Think of how laughter affects you physically and emotionally. When my mood is crabby and dark, hearing one of my daughter's big old belly laughs lightens it considerably. Have you ever noticed how a good bout of laughter dissolves stress? All the tension coursing through the nervous system gets drawn right into the solar plexus, where it is released into that distinctive sound of joy we call laughter.

The spirit of laughter is particularly evident in young children. Adults often try to tap into it. Watch kid-crazy grandparents standing behind a baby or a toddler in a checkout line. They wave, point, waggle their fingers, and make silly faces as they try to coax a smile or giggle out of the child. Regardless of age, every spirit is lifted by laughter, and even by a sincere smile. Of course, we need healing tears and frowns, but we also need to let loose and get loose with some big old belly laughs.

Fifteen-month-old Hannah and I were playing outside with a ball. I tossed it to her and she tried to catch it. I moved very close to her and rolled the ball around her tummy. She threw the ball and started laughing. I picked it up and gently pushed it into her tummy again. She threw it and laughed harder. Pretty soon this miniature person was weaving around the grass drunk with laughter, making me laugh, too. Wouldn't it be better than a hot fudge sundae if we could laugh like that every day?

Nature

Like laughter, nature speaks directly to our spirits. No translation is required. We instinctively know that a geranium-pink sunset soothes our tired shoulders and that the air after a summer rainstorm sparkles in our nostrils. Of all the animals in the kingdom, only humans behold beauty. We see it through our spirits. We have a need for beauty and nature in our lives. When I asked my friend what he had done over the weekend, he replied that he and his wife had taken a walk in a nearby canyon "just to see something beautiful." Have you ever needed a nature fix? If I work too long indoors, I crave fresh air and plants and birds. The still waters of nature restore the human soul.

Children gravitate to the outdoors. A classic toddler pose is to stand with her nose pressed against the screen door, chanting "Out! Out!" Nature tempts our senses; and children, being so sensate, revel in the touch, taste, smell, sound, and sight of their natural environment. Think of your own childhood memories. When I went to my high school reunion, my best friend from sixth grade and I reminisced about the fort we had built in the field near our houses. Next to our bark-assembled lean-to was an old tree limb that was like a carnival ride when we got it bouncing just the right way. The feel of that limb, the smell of the clay earth, and the sound of the whispering wheat are all indelibly etched in my memory. Our children need to record their own memories for future inspiration and tranquility.

One day our doorbell rang. Tristan, one of the three neighborhood kids playing on the driveway, asked for a container in which to capture grasshoppers. Southern Arizona breeds grasshoppers big enough to be household pets. I scrounged up a plastic box with a lid that had originally stored crayons and paints. It was not designed to hold anything requiring oxygen.

A short time later the front door opened and in burst Tristan.

"Miss Lynn," exclaimed the five-year-old, almost in tears. "The grasshopper can't breathe. He's jumping against the sides and scratching to get out." His little hands swam through the air.

He described the grasshopper so well that I could almost feel the poor thing gasping for air. I wondered if he really could feel the grasshopper's discomfort, just like a mother feels the pain of her child's freshly skinned knee. He was hesitant to lift the lid, afraid the two older children would berate him. We went outside, and I lifted the lid off the box. Tristan sighed with relief as the long, graceful insect jumped out and hopped across the stone-covered yard into the desert.

Oh, that we could all learn to feel and ease nature's pains.

Faith

What is faith?

How many times have people struggled to answer this question? In the most general sense, faith is a personal awareness of our connection to a universal benevolence, a glory, an enduring love that permeates everything. This love has many names: God, Goddess, Universe, Divine Spirit, the Absolute, Yahweh, Gaia. Regardless of what term you use—I'll use "God"—faith is a personal viewpoint of the interconnectedness of people, nature, Earth, solar systems, and the universe.

Faith is inborn. It is not a product of organized religion although religion certainly can foster faith. Children enter this world with the seeds of faith implanted in their spirits. When cared for properly, these seeds sprout and blossom into a deeper awareness of God's presence in the world. This awareness serves as a security base, solid and strong. It's the permanent rock we stand on as life's inevitable trials undulate around us.

What if those seeds aren't watered or the stem of faith shrivels? In a life without faith, a person feels isolated and vulnerable. Sure, there may be connections to family and friends, and perhaps to a job, an income, and material things. These things can serve as one's security and measure of self-worth. But because these connections are temporary and flimsy, the world appears to be as fragile as life itself. Faith, on the other hand, connects us with a power—a force, a universe, a God—that is enduring and everlasting. Through faith, we relate to God.

Six-year-old Elle and I were savoring the green grass of a playground during a summer visit to Wisconsin. The big maple tree near us brought to my mind memories of first grade and maple trees and little maple-seed helicopters. My children know saguaro cactus and prickly pears. Living in the desert, they do not know maple trees.

"Look, Elle," I said, picking up one of the maple seeds. "When you throw these up in the air, they spin down like a helicopter." I threw it up and we watched the seed twirl down to the ground.

After a few dozen seed choppers went flying through the air, we sat down again. Elle looked contemplatively at the stately tree that had shared its treasures with us. I started to point out other trees—birch, oak, elm.

"Does God live everywhere?" she asked. Okay, I thought, time to move on from the subject of trees.

"Yes, honey," I said, "God lives everywhere."

"Does He live in the maple helicopters?"

"Yes, I suppose He even lives in the maple helicopters."

She paused for a moment.

"Does He get dizzy in there?"

The Practice of Faith

The statement "I have faith" implies a belief in a higher power. Faith, when practiced, connects us to this higher power. You may philosophically understand a discipline such as tai chi or yoga, or have training in herbal medicine or homeopathy, but what benefit are these teachings if you don't put them to use? Faith is similar. Unattended, it lies fallow. It serves us best when we actively use it. In other words, we must practice faith. Once we get an inkling of the divine nature of life, our faith is awakened. A natural response to this awakening is a desire to connect to divinity, be it in a formal way through organized religion or in a personal manner.

Acts of faith come in different shapes and forms. Prayer is one form. A prayer can be a five-second thought that addresses God or it can be said aloud and in unison by a congregation during a church service. For children, prayer is not an intellectual endeavor or challenge; rather, it provides the opportunity to participate. It appeals to that part of a child's spirit that needs to relate actively to life in some ultimate and greater sense. Just as children perceive the interconnectedness of life through nature, they will also begin to comprehend it through the actions of liturgy. Acts of faith lead us to the grander and healthier whole universe that lies beyond our fragmented society.

Every child, whether raised as a Christian, Jew, Buddhist, Muslim, Hindu, or otherwise has a spirit and, as such, is connected to Spirit. Parents are responsible for caring for their child's spirit, that very heart of being. What an awesome, utterly wonderful, and cherished responsibility and experience that is. Because as the child grows, so must the parent.

Epilogue

June 2000

As usual, the school bus stopped at our house promptly at 3:30 P.M. A minute later, Elle walked through the front door crying. This was not her usual disposition upon returning from school.

"My ear hurts," she said through tears, holding a hand over her left ear. "It's really bad."

That morning she awakened with a terribly stuffy nose. I gave her the tissue remedy Kali sulph., but since she didn't have a sore throat or a fever and appeared chipper, I sent her to school. An hour before school ended, the earache started and grew progressively painful.

Neither of the girls had ever had an ear infection with a sharp, stitching pain. In fact, it was an acute illness that made me particularly nervous. Watching my child suffer through pain is much more difficult for me than watching her suffer through a stuffy nose, fever, sore throat, cold, vomiting, or stomachache. We already had dealt with those situations. Homeopathy had always helped cure them. Could I trust remedies to heal Elle's ear pain within a reasonable amount of time?

The day before, I had completed the chart on tissue remedies that you saw at the end of chapter 5. My inclination was to call our homeopath to confirm that I should use Ferrum phos., as listed on the chart. More than anything, I needed a little hand-holding. I was nervous as I watched Elle move restlessly on the couch, clearly in pain. I remembered the discomfort of that inner ear pain from my childhood.

I knew that our homeopath had left town for the weekend and couldn't be reached. Gregg, my moral support and second opinion, was away until early evening. I felt like the Lone Ranger, with our Siamese cat as Tonto.

The alternative to homeopathy, of course, was to take this hurting child to an emergency room or urgent care clinic. This would entail driving in rush hour traffic on a 100-degree day. I estimated two to three hours before I would have antibiotic in hand. I opted for the Ferrum phos.

"Okay, Elle," I said. "This remedy works really well on ear infections."

I gave her two tablets of Ferrum phos. 6x every fifteen minutes. Between doses, I rubbed her legs, read her a fairy tale, and anxiously flitted around doing menial chores. After an hour, she announced that the pain had lessened. Then she fell asleep. I breathed easier.

About an hour later, she awoke. Her ear still hurt, she said, but not too bad. I gave her another dose of Ferrum phos. By the time she went to bed, the pain had disappeared, although she still looked a tad pale.

You can surmise all sorts of explanations for her recovery. Homeopathy is an excellent placebo. Homeopathy is excellent medicine. Homeopathy is nothing but sugar pills; the earache resolved itself. In any case, the remedy worked, and I felt as triumphant as Rocky Balboa climbing up those stairs. I trusted homeopathy and, despite the nervous ball in my stomach, trusted myself to use the remedies correctly. If the remedies had not worked, I would have consulted a medical professional. As it turned out, I didn't need to do that. The experience boosted my confidence in my ability to handle acute illness.

The next day, I had an opportunity to relive the experience. Hannah's friend Jacque spent the afternoon at our house and the girls finagled a sleepover. At about 8:00 P.M., I noticed Hannah mixing our family's standard sore throat treatment: 2 teaspoons salt mixed in a glass of warm water with a pinch of turmeric, an antibacterial, added.

"Jacque has a sore throat, Mama," Hannah told me. I also gave Jacque two Ferrum phos. tablets. We know Jacque's family well, and I knew that giving her the medicine wasn't going to cause a stir.

Everyone soon settled into bed. Just before midnight, Hannah shook me awake.

"Mama, Jacque's crying. Her ear hurts."

Again? Did someone rewind the video and insert a new actor in the lead role? Poor Jacque. She looked as uncomfortable as Elle had the day before. I retrieved the Ferrum phos. and went through the same motion of two tablets every fifteen minutes. Once again, the pain subsided, this time after an hour and a quarter. Jacque fell asleep soundly and in the morning was jumping around like nothing had happened.

Will Ferrum phos. help cure every ear infection with sharp pain? I'm not sure anyone can offer that guarantee. Nevertheless, at a time when antibiotics are losing their effectiveness, isn't the remedy worth a try, particularly since it has no side effects?

If we parents became adept at using home remedies for the inevitable acute illnesses of life, would doctors have more time to spend with patients suffering from chronic illness? Would emergency rooms be less burdened during cold and flu season? Would antibiotics be more trustworthy for serious acute conditions like pneumonia and meningitis?

Over the years, my family's lifestyle has become increasingly natural. When someone contracts a common acute illness, we don't run to the doctor. We first turn to the medicine cabinet or spice cabinet for a homeopathic or herbal remedy. Illnesses don't seem to last as long as they used to last. From the cleaning cabinet, we have eliminated toxic liquids, powders, and creams. Most of our foods are organic. To some extent, our lifestyle seems simpler. Perhaps this is because nature, in spite of her complexities, is simple. When we follow the laws of nature, we eliminate complications and side effects induced by the artificial and the synthetic. Consequently, we thrive.

This holistic natural living affords us more than healthy bodies. If allowed to flourish, a holistic lifestyle imbues us with a sense of wonder, joy, and gratitude. The challenge for each of us lies in allowing ourselves to change our attitudes and viewpoints and to experiment with new ideas and medicines. As we accumulate experiences and traverse new ground, our confidence grows. We begin to teach others. Like the ripples that spread around a single drop of water on a placid lake, the ripples of change encircle more and more people.

Physicist Max Planck said, "A new scientific truth does not triumph by convincing its opponents and making them see the light, but rather because its opponents eventually die, and a new generation grows up that is familiar with it." Being a parent, I am no longer of the "new" generation, but this does not mean that I must remain ignorant. I have decided to learn and change and to teach my children along the way. For me, that process is part of the whole of life. For you, dear reader, it may or may not be the same. You must decide.

God bless you on your journey.

NOTES

Chapter 1

1. Clayton L. Thomas, M.D., ed. *Taber's Cyclopedic Medical Dictionary* (Philadelphia: Davis Co., 1993).

2. Amanda Spake. "Losing the Battle of the Bugs." *U.S. News & World Report* (May 10, 1999).

3. Elena Portyansky. "Antibiotic Resistance Is Fueled by Community Overprescribing." *Drug Topics* 124, No. 4 (February 16, 1998): 34.

4. Jason Lazarou, M.Sc., et al. "Incidence of Adverse Drug Reactions in Hospitalized Patients: A Meta-Analysis of Prospective Studies." *Journal of the American Medical Association* 279, No. 15 (April 15, 1998): 1200–1205.

5. Jane Everhart. "Antibiotic Overuse and Misuse Linked to Bacterial Resistance." *American Druggist* 216, No. 4 (April 1, 1999): 21.

6. Spake, "Losing the Battle."

7. Everhart, "Antibiotic Overuse."

8. David Eisenberg, M.D., et al. "Unconventional Medicine in the United States: Prevalence, Costs, and Patterns of Use." *Journal of the American Medical Association* 328, No. 4 (January 28, 1993): 246–252.

9. Harriet Beinfield, L.Ac. and Efrem Korngold, L.Ac. *Between Heaven and Earth: A Guide to Chinese Medicine* (New York: Ballantine Books, 1991).

Chapter 2

1. L. S. Barden, et al. "Current Attitudes Regarding Use of Antimicrobial Agents: Results from Physicians' and Parents' Focus Group Discussions." *Clinical Pediatrics* (November 1998): 665–672.

2. Rebecca L. Watson, et al. "Antimicrobial Use for Pediatric Upper Respiratory Infections: Reported Practice, Actual Practice, and Parent Belief." *Journal of the American Medical Association* 283, No. 5 (February 2000): 586.

3. Jennifer Couzen. "Cleaning Up: Battling Bugs in the Home." *U.S. News & World Report* (May 10, 1999).

4. Ann M. Arvin, M.D. "Live Attenuated Varicella Vaccine." *Pediatric Annals* 26, No. 6 (June 1997): 384–388.

5. Mona Lisa Schulz, M.D., Ph.D. *Awakening Intuition* (New York: Harmony Books, 1998).

6. David Russell. *Names of Life* (Unpublished, 1999).

7. Eric Cassell. *The Nature of Suffering* (New York: Oxford University Press, 1991).

Chapter 3

1. Julian Scott, Ph.D. "The Treatment of Children by Acupuncture." *Journal of Chinese Medicine* (1986).

2. Henry Skolimowski, Ph.D. "Wholeness, Hippocrates, and Ancient Philosophy." In *Spiritual Healing,* Dora Kunz, ed. (Wheaton, Ill.: The Theosophical Publishing House, 1995).

3. Hippocrates. *On Airs, Waters, and Places.* http://classics.mit.edu/Hippocrates/airwatpl.1.1.html (4 April, 1999).

4. Dr. Wighard Strehlow and Gottfried Hertzka, M.D. *Hildegard of Bingen's Medicine.* Trans. Karin Anderson Strehlow (Santa Fe: Bear & Company, Inc., 1988).

5. Fritjof Capra. *The Turning Point: Science, Society, and the Rising Culture* (New York: Bantam Books, 1982).

6. Thomas S. Kuhn. *The Structure of Scientific Revolutions* (Chicago: University of Chicago Press, 1962).

Chapter 4

1. Julian Scott, Ph.D. *Natural Medicine for Children* (New York: Avon Books, 1990).

2. Nicholas Culpeper. *The English Physician;* and *Complete Herbal: A Basic of Natural Remedies for Ancient Ills* (London: Champante and Whitrow, 1789).

3. Rosemary Gladstar. *Herbal Remedies for Children's Health* (Pownal, VT: Storey Books, 1999).

Chapter 5

1. Dana Ullman, M.P.H. *Homeopathic Medicine for Children and Infants* (New York: G. P. Putnam's Sons, 1992).

2. Ullman, *Discovering Homeopathy: Medicine for the 21st Century* (Berkeley, Calif.: North Atlantic Books, 1991).

3. Rick Chillot. "Homeopathy: Help or Hype?" *Prevention,* March, 1998.

4. "Homeopathy Gains Additional Converts." *Chain Drug Review,* October 6, 1997.

5. Dana Ullman, M.P.H. *The Consumer's Guide to Homeopathy* (New York: Jeremy P. Tarcher/Putnam, 1995).

6. Jan P. Vandenbroucke. "Homeopathy Trials: Going Nowhere." *Lancet* 350, No. 9081 (September 20, 1997): 824.

7. Varro E. Tyler, Ph.D., Sc.D., *The Honest Herbal: A Sensible Guide to the Use of Herbs and Related Remedies* (New York: Pharmaceutical Products Press, 1992).

8. K. H. Friese, et al. "Acute Otitis Media in Children: A Comparison of Conventional and Homeopathic Treatment." *Biomedical Therapy* 60, No. 4 (August 1996): 462–66.

9. Jennifer Jacobs, et al. "Treatment of Acute Childhood Diarrhea with Homeopathic Medicine: A Randomized Clinical Trial in Nicaragua." *Pediatrics* 93, No. 5 (May 1994): 719–25.

10. J. Kleijnen, et al. "Clinical Trials of Homeopathy." *British Medical Journal* 302 (February 9, 1991): 316–323.

11. Klaus Linde, et al. "Are the Clinical Effects of Homeopathy Placebo Effects? A Meta-Analysis of Placebo-Controlled Trials." *Lancet* 350, No. 9081 (September 20, 1997): 834–843.

12. Judyth Reichenberg-Ullman and Robert Ullman. *Ritalin-Free Kids: Safe and Effective Homeopathic Medicine for ADD and Other Behavioral and Learning Problems.* (Rocklin, Calif.: Prima Publishing, 1996.)

13. George Vithoulkas. *The Science of Homeopathy* (New York: Grove Press, Inc., 1980).

14. Ullman, *Homeopathic Medicine for Children and Infants.*

Chapter 6

1. G. Lubec, C. Wolf, and B. Bartosch. "Aminoacid Isomerisation and Microwave Exposure," *Lancet,* December 9, 1989: 1392–1393.

2. David Frawley, O.M.D. *Ayurvedic Healing: A Comprehensive Guide* (Salt Lake City: Passage Press, 1989).

Chapter 7

1. Eileen Kennedy, D.Sc., R.D. and Jeanne Goldberg, Ph.D., R.D. "What Are American Children Eating? Implications for Public Policy." *Nutrition Reviews* 53, No. 5 (May 1995): 111–126.

2. Michael F. Jacobson, Ph.D. and Bruce Maxwell. *What Are We Feeding Our Kids?* (New York: Workman Publishing, 1994).

3. Annemarie Colbin. *Food and Healing* (New York: Ballantine Books, 1986).

4. Alan Reder, Phil Catalfo, and Stephanie Renfrow Hamilton. *The Whole Parenting Guide* (New York: Broadway Books, 1999).

5. Paul Pitchford. *Healing with Whole Foods: Oriental Traditions and Modern Nutrition* (Berkeley, Calif.: North Atlantic Books, 1993).

6. Colbin, *Food and Healing.*

7. Jane Brody. "Diet Change May Avert Need for Ritalin." *New York Times,* November 2, 1999.

8. Center for Science in the Public Interest. "Scientists' Letters to the Department of Health and Human Services." October 25, 1999, http://www.cspinet.org/new/adhdletters.html (27 March 2000).

9. Center for Science in the Public Interest, "Scientists' Letters to the Department of Health and Human Services."

10. Nancy Gibbs. "The Age of Ritalin." *Time,* November 30, 1998.

11. Doris J. Rapp, M.D. *Is This Your Child's World?* (New York: Bantam Books, 1996).

12. Wolrach, Mark L., M.D., David B. Wilson, Ph.D., and J. Wade White, M.D. "The Effect of Sugar on Behavior or Cognition in Children: A Meta-Analysis." *Journal of the American Medical Association* 274, No. 20 (November 22/29, 1995): 1617–1621.

13. Colbin, *Food and Healing.*

14. Leila Corcoran and Michael Jacobson. "Saccharin: Bittersweet." *Nutrition Action Healthletter* 25, No. 3:11.

15. Mary Nash Stoddard. *Deadly Deception: Story of Aspartame* (Dallas: Oldenwald Press, 1998).

16. Stoddard, *Deadly Deception*.

17. Stoddard, *Deadly Deception*.

18. Stoddard, personal communication, June 2000.

19. Pitchford, *Healing with Whole Foods*.

20. "Food Myth #1: If It's in the Store, It Must Be Okay." The Doctor's Medical Library 1999. http://www.medical-library.net/sites/_food_myth_1.html (20 September 1999).

21. "BGH-Free Milk." Genewatch, http:/www.gene-watch.org/genewatch/genefeb.html (17 February 2000).

22. Masanobu Fukuoka. *The Natural Way of Farming: The Theory and Practice of Green Philosophy* (Tokyo: Japan Publications, 1985).

23. "Seeds of Change." *Consumer Reports,* September 1999, 41–46.

24. Laura Ticciati and Robin Ticciati, Ph.D. *Genetically Engineered Foods: Are They Safe? You Decide* (Los Angeles: Keats Publishing, 1998).

25. Ticciati, *Genetically Engineered Foods*.

26. Council for Agricultural Science and Technology. "Radiation Pasteurization of Food." April 1996, http://www.cast-science.org/past_ip.htm (15 February 2000).

27. Colbin, *Food and Healing*.

Chapter 8

1. Doris J. Rapp, M.D. *Is This Your Child's World?* (New York: Bantam Books, 1996).

2. Mark R. Sneller, Ph.D. *A Household Manual for Better Respiratory Health* (Self-published: 1998).

3. Environmental Protection Agency. *The Inside Story: A Guide to Indoor Air Quality.* EPA Document #402-K-93-007, 1995.

4. Sneller, *A Household Manual for Better Respiratory Health.*

5. Mindy Pennybacker and Aisha Ikramuddin. *Mothers & Others for a Liveable Planet's Guide to Natural Baby Care* (New York: John Wiley & Sons, Inc., 1999).

6. Rapp, *Is This Your Child's World?*

7. Environmental Protection Agency. "Organic Gases." *Sources of Information on Indoor Air Quality,* http://www.epa.gov/iaq/voc.html (1 February 2000).

8. Pennybacker, *Guide to Natural Baby Care.*

9. Sneller, *A Household Manual for Better Respiratory Health.*

10. Debra Lynn Dadd. *Nontoxic, Natural, & Earthwise* (Los Angeles: Jeremy P. Tarcher, Inc., 1990).

11. Mindy Pennybacker, ed. "Kids' Vulnerability to Pesticides." *The Green Guide,* No. 44, September 14, 1997.

12. Anonymous: "Clinical Ecology: Executive Committee of the American Academy of Allergy and Immunology". *Journal of Allergy and Clinical Immunology,* Sept 1986: 269.

13. Rapp, *Is This Your Child's World?*

Chapter 9

1. Neil Z. Miller. "Vaccines and Natural Health." *Mothering,* No. 70, Spring (1994): 48–49.

2. Centers for Disease Control and Prevention. Fax Information Services, 1997.

3. Hillary Rodham Clinton. *It Takes A Village* (New York: Simon & Schuster, 1996).

4. Harris L. Coulter and Barbara Loe Fisher. *A Shot in the Dark* (New York: Avery Publishing Group, 1991).

5. Barbara Loe Fisher. *The Consumer's Guide to Childhood Vaccines* (Vienna, Virginia: The National Vaccine Information Center, 1997).

6. Sir Arthur S. MacNalty. "The Prevention of Smallpox: From Edward Jenner to Mockton Copeman." *British Medical Journal* 2 vol. 519, no. 946 (1966): 8.

7. Scheibner, Viera, Ph.D. *Vaccination: The Medical Assault on the Immune System* (Blackheath, NSW, Australia: V. Scheibner, 1993).

8. Coulter and Fisher, *A Shot in the Dark.*

9. "Review of the First International Public Conference on Vaccination." *Mothering,* No. 86, Jan./Feb. (1998).

10. Dorothy Shepherd, M.D. *Homeopathy in Epidemic Diseases* (Rustington, Essex, U.K.: Health Sciences Press, 1967).

11. Neil Z. Miller. *Vaccines: Are They Really Safe and Effective?* (Santa Fe, New Mexico: New Atlantean Press, 1994).

12. Paul A. Offit, M.D. and Louis M. Bell, M.D. *What Every Parent Should Know About Vaccines* (New York: Macmillan, 1998).

13. Offit and Bell, *What Every Parent Should Know About Vaccines.*

14. S. A. Halperin, et al. "Persistence of Pertussis in an Immunised Population: Results of the Nova Scotia Enhanced Pertussis Surveillance Program," *Journal of Pediatrics* 1125: 686–693 (cited in Scheibner, *Vaccination.*)

15. Sir Graham Wilson. *The Hazards of Immunization* (London: The Athlone Press, 1967). As cited in Murphy, Jamie. *What Every Parent Should Know About Childhood Immunization.* (Boston, Massachusetts: Earth Healing Products, 1995.)

16. Dalya Guris, M.D., M.P.H., et al. "Pertussis Vaccination in the United States—New Developments and Recommendations." *Pediatric Annals* 26, No.6 (June 1997): 374.

17. Annemarie Colbin, *Food and Healing* (New York: Ballantine, 1996).

18. Randall Neustaedter, O.M.D. *The Vaccine Guide: Making an Informed Choice* (Berkeley Calif.: North Atlantic Books, 1996).

19. Miller, *Vaccines: Are They Really Safe and Effective?*

20. *Morbidity and Mortality Weekly Report* (MMWR) 45, No. RR-12 (September 6, 1996): 2.

21. Neustaedter, *The Vaccine Guide: Making an Informed Choice.*

22. Miller, Neil Z. "Vaccines and Natural Health." *Mothering:* 48–49.

23. Neustaedter, *The Vaccine Guide.*

24. Stanley A. Plotkin, M.D. and Edward A. Mortimer, M.D., eds. *Vaccines* (Philadelphia: W. B. Saunders Co., 1988).

25. Robert S. Mendelsohn, M.D. *How to Raise a Healthy Child . . . in Spite of Your Doctor* (New York: Ballantine Books, 1984).

26. Marcea Weber. *Encyclopedia of Natural Health and Healing for Children* (East Roseville, Australia: Simon & Schuster, 1992).

27. Michael Alderson. *International Mortality Statistics* (Washington, D.C.: Facts on File, 1981):177–178 (cited in Miller, *Vaccines*).

28. Lynne McTaggart. "The MMR Vaccine," in *Vaccinations: The Rest of the Story* (Santa Fe, New Mexico: Mothering, 2d ed., 1996).

29. Miller, *Vaccines.*

30. N. P. Thompson, et al. "Is Measles Vaccination a Risk Factor for Inflammatory Bowel Disease?" *Lancet* 345 (April 29, 1995): 1071–74.

31. Mendelsohn, *How to Raise a Healthy Child . . . in Spite of Your Doctor.*

32. Scheibner, *Vaccination.*

33. Benjamin Spock, M.D. and Michael B. Rothenberg, M.D. *Dr. Spock's Baby and Child Care* (New York: Pocket Books, 1985, 40th ed.).

34. Fisher, *The Consumer's Guide to Childhood Vaccines.*

35. Randall Neustaedter, O.M.D. *The Immunization Decision: A Guide for Parents.* (Berkeley, Calif.: North Atlantic Books, 1990).

36. Neustaedter, *The Immunization Decision.*

37. Kristine Severyn, Ph.D., ed. *Ohio Parents for Vaccine Safety Newsletter.* September 1997.

38. C. W. Jungeblut and E. T. Engle. "Resistant to Poliomylitis: The Relative Importance of Physiological and Immunological Factors." *Journal of the American Medical Association* 99, No. 25 (1932): 2091–2097.

39. Miller, "Vaccines and Natural Health."

40. Leon Chaitow, M.D. *Vaccination and Immunisation: Dangers, Delusions, and Alternatives* (Essex, England: The C. W. Daniel Company Limited, 5th ed., 1994).

41. Fisher, *The Consumer's Guide to Childhood Vaccines.*

42. Scheibner, *Vaccination.*

43. Burton Waisbren, Sr., M.D. "Universal Hepatitis B Vaccinations." *Wisconsin Medical Journal* (March 1996): 148.

44. Neustaedter, *The Vaccine Guide.*

45. Conversation with Burton Waisbren, Sr., M.D. February 4, 1998.

46. Burton A. Waisbren, Sr., M.D. "The Experiment of Universal Hepatitis B Vaccination." *Medical Crossfire.* http://www.medicalcrossfire.com/debate_archive/March _oo/HepatitisB.htm. (8 May 2000).

47. Neustaedter, *The Vaccine Guide.*

48. Neustaedter, *The Vaccine Guide.*

49. Fisher, *The Consumer's Guide to Childhood Vaccines.*

50. Ann M. Arvin. "Live Attenuated Varicella Vaccine." *Pediatric Annals* 26, No. 6 June 1997): 384–88.

51. Stephen R. Prelud, M.D. "Varicella: Complications and Costs." *Pediatrics,* Supplement (1986): 728.

52. Fisher, *The Consumer's Guide to Childhood Vaccines.*

53. William A. Altemeier, M.D. "Take Your Tricks Where You See Them." *Pediatric Annals* 26, No. 6 (June 1997): 345.

54. Scheibner, *Vaccination.*

55. Scheibner, *Vaccination.*

56. Richard Moskowitz, M.D. "Unvaccinated Children" in *Vaccinations: The Rest of the Story* (Santa Fe, New Mexico: Mothering, 2nd ed., 1996).

57. Fisher, *The Consumer's Guide to Childhood Vaccines.*

58. Coulter and Fisher, *A Shot in the Dark.*

59. Fisher, *The Consumer's Guide to Childhood Vaccines.*

Chapter 10

1. Mark A. Breiner, D.D.S. *Whole-Body Dentistry: Discover the Missing Piece to Better Health* (Fairfield, CT: Quantum Health Press, 1999).

2. Michael Downey. "A Crack Appears in the Fluoride Front." *Toronto Star,* April 25, 1999.

3. American Dental Association. "Fluoridation Facts." 1999. http://www.ada.org/consumer/fluoride/facts/benefits.html.

4. Susan Duerksen. "Staining of Teeth on Increase in Treated, Nontreated Areas." *San Diego Union-Tribune,* Sept. 1, 1999.

5. Dana Canady. "Toothpaste a Hazard? Just Ask the FDA." *New York Times,* March 24, 1998.

6. "Dentists Fear Hidden Cost of Bottled Water." *New York Times,* November 3, 1998.

7. Dr. John Yiamouyiannis. *Fluoride the Aging Factor: How to Recognize and Avoid the Devastating Effects of Fluoride* (Delaware, Ohio: Health Action Press, 1986).

8. Yiamouyiannis, *Fluoride the Aging Factor.*

9. Yiamouyiannis, *Fluoride the Aging Factor.*

10. Yiamouyiannis, *Fluoride the Aging Factor.*

11. Yiamouyiannis, *Fluoride the Aging Factor.*

12. "Fluoride May Be Linked to Brain Tissue Damage." *Medical Industry Today,* 20 April 1998.

13. "Fluoride May Be Linked to Brain Tissue Damage." *Medical Industry Today.*

14. David R. Hill. "Fluoride: Risks and Benefits?" August 1997. http://www.cadvision.com/fluoride/calgaryh.html.

15. P. D. Cohn. "A Brief Report on the Association of Drinking Water Fluoridation and the Incidence of Osteosarcoma Among Young Males." New Jersey Department of Health (Trenton, New Jersey: November 1992).

16. Yiamouyiannis, *Fluoride the Aging Factor.*

17. Citizens for Safe Drinking Water. "Dangers of Fluoridated Water." http://www.nofluoride.com (21 May 2000).

18. Citizens for Safe Drinking Water, "Dangers of Fluoridated Water."

19. International Society for Fluoride Research. *Fluoride.* http://www.fluoride-journal.com (13 December 1999).

20. Downey, "A Crack Appears in the Fluoride Front."

21. American Dental Association. "Dental Amalgam: 150 Years of Safety and Effectiveness." ADA News Releases, November 1995. http://www.ada.org/newsrel/1195/nr-02a.html (13 December 1999).

22. Sam Ziff and Michael F. Ziff, D.D.S. *Infertility & Birth Defects: Is Mercury from Silver Dental Fillings an Unsuspected Cause?* (Orlando: Bio-Probe, Inc., 1987).

23. Ziff, *Infertility & Birth Defects.*

24. Sam Ziff and Michael F. Ziff, D.D.S. *Dentistry Without Mercury* (Orlando: Bio-Probe, Inc., 1997).

25. Ziff, *Infertility & Birth Defects*.

26. Hal A. Huggins, D.D.S., M.S. *It's All in Your Head: The Link Between Mercury Amalgams and Illness* (Garden City Park, N.Y.: Avery Publishing Group, Inc., 1993).

27. Huggins, *It's All in Your Head*.

28. James E. Hardy, D.D.S. *Mercury Free: The Wisdom Behind the Global Consumer Movement to Ban "Silver" Dental Fillings* (Glassboro, NJ: Gabriel Rose Press, Inc., 1996).

Chapter 11

1. Kurt Butler. *The Consumer's Guide to Alternative Medicine: A Close Look at Homeopathy, Acupuncture, Faith-Healing, and Other Unconventional Treatments* (Buffalo: Prometheus Books, 1992).

2. "Quotations by Galileo Galilei." http://www-groups.dcs.st-and.ac.uk/~history/Quotations/Galileo.html (18 January 2000).

3. Mary Chris Jakleui. "Physician Compensation Growth Slows." *Modern Healthcare*, August 2, 1999.

4. Michelle Andrews. "The Doctor Will See Your Soul Now." *Smart Money*, December 1999.

5. "What is a Skeptic?" *Skeptic* 6., no. 2 (1998): 5.

6. National Council Against Health Fraud. "Position Paper on Homeopathy." http://www.hcrc.org/ncahf/pos-pap/homeop.html (9 January 2000).

7. "Acupuncture Laws by State." http://www.acupuncture.com/StateLaws/StateLaws.htm (29 January, 2000).

Chapter 12

1. Thomas Moore. *Care of the Soul* (New York: HarperPerennial, 1994).

2. Richard Lewis. *Living by Wonder: The Imaginative Life of Childhood* (New York: Parabola Books, 1998).

3. Jane Healy, Ph.D. "Understanding TV's Effects on the Developing Brain." (http://www.aap.org./advocacy/chm98nws.htm (21 March 2000).

4. Julian Scott, Ph.D. "The Treatment of Children by Acupuncture." *Journal of Chinese Medicine* (1986).

5. American Academy of Pediatrics. "Smart Guide to Kids' TV." http://www.aap.org./family/smarttv.htm (21 March 2000).

6. Kondrake, Morton. "Don't Kill Your TV to Reduce Total Viewing Hours, Just Bind and Gag It." *Arizona Daily Star,* August 30, 1997.

BIBLIOGRAPHY

Chapter 1

Astin, John A., Ph.D. "Why Patients Use Alternative Medicine: Results of a National Study." *Journal of the American Medical Association* 279, no. 19 (May 20, 1998): 1548–1553.

Cassell, Eric. *The Nature of Suffering and the Goals of Medicine.* New York: Oxford University Press, 1991.

Carlson, Katherine. "Body and Soul: Alternative Medicine— University of Minnesota Center for Spirituality and Healing." *Minneapolis-St. Paul Magazine* 26, no. 10 (October 1998): 102.

Chopra, Deepak, M.D. *Quantum Healing: Exploring the Frontiers of Mind/Body Medicine.* New York: Bantam Books, 1989.

Dacher, Elliot, M.D. "The Whole Healing System." 1996. http://www.healthy.net/dacher/whs.htm (21 August 1998).

Eisenberg, David, M.D., et al. "Unconventional Medicine in the United States: Prevalence, Costs, and Patterns of Use." *Journal of the American Medical Association* 328, no. 4 (1993): 246–252.

"Fiscal Year 2000 President's Budget Request for NCCAM." http://nccam.nih.gov/nccam/news-events/press-releases/1.htm (3 May 1999).

Gaedeke, Ralph, et al. "Alternative Therapies: Familiarity, Use, and Information Needs." *Marketing Health Services,* Summer 1999.

Integrative Medicine Program Seminar. Tucson, Arizona. May 8, 1999.

Kunz, Dora, ed. *Spiritual Healing: Doctors Examine Therapeutic Touch and Other Holistic Treatments.* Wheaton, Ill.: The Theosophical Publishing House, 1985.

Lazarou, Jason, M.Sc., et al. "Incidence of Adverse Drug Reactions in Hospitalized Patients: A Meta-Analysis of Prospective Studies." *Journal of the American Medical Association* 279, no. 15 (April 15, 1998): 1200–1205.

Mendelsohn, Robert S., M.D. *Confessions of a Medical Heretic.* Chicago: Contemporary Books, 1979.

Spiegel, David, et al. "Complementary Medicine." *Western Journal of Medicine* 168, no. 4 (April 1998).

"Survey: Alternative Therapies Complement Traditional Care." *Medical Industry Today,* August 19, 1999.

Thomas, Clayton, L., M.D., ed. *Taber's Cyclopedic Medical Dictionary.* Philadelphia: Davis Co., 1993.

Weil, Andrew, M.D. *Health and Healing.* New York: Houghton Mifflin Company, 1983.

Zand, Janet, L.Ac., O.M.D., Rachel Walton, R.N., and Bob Roundtree, M.D. *Smart Medicine for a Healthier Child: A Practical A to Z Reference to Natural and Conventional Treatments for Infants and Children.* Garden City Park, NY: Avery Publishing Group, 1994.

Zintl, Amy. "Natural Cures for Kids; Alternative Medicine for Children." *Ladies Home Journal,* October 1998; 56.

Chapter 2

"Antibiotic Attitudes." *Child Health Alert,* January 1999.

"Are Doctors Changing the Way They Treat Ear Infections?" *Child Health Alert,* May 1, 1999.

Cassell, Eric. *The Nature of Suffering.* New York: Oxford University Press, 1991.

Dubos, Rene. *Mirage of Health.* New York: Harper, 1959.

Everhart, Jane. "Antibiotic Overuse and Misuse Linked to Bacterial Resistance." *American Druggist,* April 1, 1999.

Finger, Anne L. "When Should Patients Have the Last Word?" *Medical Economics,* June 15, 1998.

Ince, Susan. "Killer Bacteria: All You've Got to Know to Stay Safe." *Redbook,* April, 1998.

Krishnamurti, J. *On Fear.* New York: HarperSanFrancisco, 1995.

Portyansky, Elena. "Antibiotic Resistance Is Fueled by Community Overprescribing." *Drug Topics,* February 16, 1998.

Schulz, Mona Lisa, M.D., Ph.D. *Awakening Intuition.* New York: Harmony Books, 1998.

Spake, Amanda. "Losing the Battle of the Bugs; Use of Antibacterial Drugs Promotes Drug-Resistant Organisms." *U.S. News & World Report,* May 10, 1999.

Tomes, Nancy. *The Gospel of Germs: Men, Women, and the Microbe in American Life.* Cambridge: Harvard University Press, 1998.

Chapter 3

Beinfield, Harriet, L.Ac. and Efrem Korngold, L.Ac., O.M.D. *Between Heaven and Earth: A Guide to Chinese Medicine.* New York: Ballantine Books, 1991.

Capra, Fritjof. *The Tao of Physics.* 3d ed. Boston: Shambhala Publications, Inc., 1991.

Capra, Fritjof. *The Turning Point: Science, Society, and the Rising Culture.* New York: Bantam Books, 1982.

Flanagan, Sabina. *Hildegard of Bingen, 1098–1179: A Visionary Life.* New York: Routledge, 1989.

Hume, Edward H. *The Chinese Way in Medicine.* Baltimore: John Hopkins Press, 1940.

Kaptchuk, Ted J., O.M.D. *The Web That Has No Weaver: Understanding Chinese Medicine.* Chicago: Congdon & Weed, Inc., 1983.

Kuhn, Thomas S. *The Structure of Scientific Revolutions.* Chicago: University of Chicago Press, 1962.

McInerney, Maud Burnett, ed. *Hildegard of Bingen: A Book of Essays.* New York: Garland Publishing, Inc., 1998.

Pernoud, Regine. *Hildegard of Bingen: Inspired Conscience of the Twelfth Century.* Trans. Paul Dugan. New York: Marlow & Co., 1998.

Porkert, Manfred. *The Theoretical Foundations of Chinese Medicine: Systems of Correspondence.* Cambridge: MIT Press, 1974.

Scott, Julian, Ph.D. "The Treatment of Children by Acupunture." *Journal of Chinese Medicine,* 1986.

Skolimowski, Henry, Ph.D. "Wholeness, Hippocrates, and Ancient Philosophy." In *Spiritual Healing,* Dora Kunz, ed. Wheaton, Ill.: The Theosophical Publishing House, 1995.

Strehlow, Wighard, Dr. and Gottfried Hertzka, M.D. *Hildegard of Bingen's Medicine.* Trans. Karin Anderson Strehlow. Santa Fe: Bear & Company, Inc., 1988.

Weil, Andrew, M.D. *Health and Healing.* Boston: Houghton Mifflin Company, 1983.

Wilber, Ken. *A Brief History of Everything.* Boston: Shambhala Publications, Inc., 1996.

Zukav, Gary. *The Dancing Wu Li Masters: An Overview of the New Physics.* New York: William Morrow, 1979.

Chapter 4

Borins, Mel, M.D., C.C.F.P. "The Dangers of Using Herbs." *Post Graduate Medicine,* 104, no. 1 (July 1998): 91.

Castleman, Michael. *The Healing Herbs: The Ultimate Guide to the Curative Power of Nature's Medicines.* Emmaus, Pa.: Rodale Press, 1991.

Cowan, Eliot. *Plant Spirit Medicine: The Healing Power of Plants.* Newberg, Oreg.: Swan-Raven, 1995.

Culpeper, Nicholas. *The English Physician;* and *Complete Herbal: A Basic of Natural Remedies for Ancient Ills.* London: Champante and Whitrow, 1789.

DiMartino, Christina. "Herbal Therapies." *Rehab Report,* August 1999.

Dodt, Colleen. *Natural BabyCare: Pure and Soothing Recipes and Techniques for Mothers and Babies.* Woodstock: Ash Tree Publishing, 1997.

Gladstar, Rosemary. *Herbal Remedies for Children's Health.* Pownal, VT: Storey Books, 1999.

Greenwald, John. "Herbal Healing." *Time,* November 23, 1998.

Griggs, Barbara. *Green Pharmacy: A History of Herbal Medicine.* London: Jill Norman & Hobhouse Ltd, 1981.

Hoffmann, David. *The Elements of Herbalism.* New York: Barnes & Noble, Inc., 1990.

Holmes, Peter. *The Energetics of Western Herbs: Integrating Western and Oriental Herbal Medicine Traditions, Volume I.* Boulder: Artemis, 1989.

Kay, Margarita Artschwager. *Healing with Plants in the American and Mexican West.* Tucson: The University of Arizona Press, 1996.

Kenner, Dan and Yves Requena. *Botanical Medicine: A European Professional Perspective.* Brookline: Paradigm Publications, 1996.

Krishnamurthy, K. H. *Ginger and Turmeric.* Delhi: Books for All, 1992.

Lawson, Larry D. and Rudolf Bauer, eds. *Phytomedicines of Europe: Chemistry and Biological Activity.* Washington, D.C.: American Chemical Society, 1998.

Moore, Michael. *Los Remedios: Traditional Herbal Remedies of the Southwest.* Santa Fe: Red Crane Books, 1990.

Nuzzi, Debra. *Pocket Herbal Reference Guide.* Freedom, Calif.: The Crossing Press, 1992.

Ody, Penelope. *Home Herbal: A Practical Guide to Making Herbal Remedies for Common Ailments.* New York: DK Publishing, Inc., 1995.

Robbers, James E., Ph.D. and Varro E. Tyler, Ph.D., Sc.D. *Tyler's Herbs of Choice: The Therapeutic Use of Phytomedicinals*. Binghamton, N.Y.: The Haworth Press, Inc., 1999.

Scott, Julian, Ph.D. *Natural Medicine for Children*. New York: Avon Books, 1990.

Sprague, Jonathan. "A Leaf from the Book of Life." *Asiaweek*, August 6, 1999.

Sturdivant, Lee and Tim Blakley. *The Bootstrap Guide to Medicinal Herbs in the Garden, Field & Marketplace*. Friday Harbor: San Juan Naturals, 1999.

"Tea for Two: Less Cancer, Less Heart Disease?" *Consumer Reports Travel Letter* 8, no. 12 (December 1996): 138–139.

Tenney, Deanne. *Aloe Vera*. Pleasant Grove, UT: Woodland Publishing, 1997.

Tierra, Michael, C.A., N.D. *Planetary Herbology*. Santa Fe: Lotus Press, 1988.

Tyler, Varro E., Ph.D., Sc.D. *The Honest Herbal: A Sensible Guide to the Use of Herbs and Related Remedies*. New York: Pharmaceutical Products Press, 1992.

Worwood, Valerie Ann. *The Complete Book of Essential Oils & Aromatherapy*. San Rafael: New World Library, 1991.

Zampieron, Eugene R, N.D., A.G.H. and Ellen Kamhi, Ph.D., R.N., H.N.C. *The Natural Medicine Chest: Natural Medicines to Keep You and Your Family Thriving into the Next Millennium*. New York: M. Evans and Company, Inc., 1999.

Chapter 5

Boericke, William and Willis Dewey. *The Twelve Tissue Remedies of Schüssler.* New Dehli: Jaine Publishers, reprint 1989.

Dolby, Victoria. " 'De-stress' the Distress in Your Child's Life with Homeopathy." *Better Nutrition,* December 1997.

Fisher, Peter. "Time to Take Homeopathy Seriously." *Chemistry and Industry,* no. 23 (December 1, 1997): 974.

Gerber, Richard. *Vibrational Medicine: New Choices for Healing Ourselves.* Sante Fe: Bear & Co., 1988.

Glissen, James, et al. "Review, Critique, and Guidelines for the Use of Herbs and Homeopathy." *Nurse Practitioner* 24, no. 4 (April 1, 1999): 44.

Gormley, James, " 'Heal Thyself': Homeopathy for a New Millennium." *Better Nutrition,* May 1998.

Hardman, Robert. "Prince Pioneers Alternative Option: Scientists May Scoff But 'Complementary' Medicine Long Championed by Kings and Queens." *Daily Telegraph,* October 21, 1997.

Langman, M. J. S. "Homeopathy Trials: Reason for Good Ones But Are They Warranted?" *Lancet* 350, no. 9081 (September 20, 1997): 825.

Lewith, George. "The Homeopathic Conundrum Revisited," *Alternative Therapies in Health and Medicine* 5, no. 5 (Sept./Oct. 1995): 32–34.

National Center for Homeopathy. "Research." http://www.healthy.net/nch/research.htm (18 August 1999).

Oh, Vernon. "The Powerful Placebo: From Ancient Priest to Modern Physician." *British Medical Journal* 316, no. 7141 (May 2, 1998).

Stehlin, Isadora. "Homeopathy: Real Medicine or Empty Promises?" *FDA Consumer* 30, no. 10 (December 1, 1996): 15.

Ullman, Dana, M.P.H. *The Consumer's Guide to Homeopathy.* New York: Jeremy P. Tarcher/Putnam, 1995.

Ullman, Dana, M.P.H. *Discovering Homeopathy: Medicine for the 21st Century.* Berkeley: North Atlantic Books, 1991.

Ullman, Dana, M.P.H. *Homeopathic Medicine for Children and Infants.* New York: G. P. Putnam's Sons, 1992.

Vandenbroucke, Jan P. "Homeopathy Trials: Going Nowhere." *Lancet* 350, no. 9081 (September 20, 1997): 824.

Vandenbroucke, Jan P. "Medical Journals and the Shaping of Medical Knowledge." *Lancet* 352, no. 9145 (December 19, 1998): 2001.

Vithoulkas, George. *The Science of Homeopathy.* New York: Grove Weidenfeld, 1980.

Chapter 6

Chopra, Deepak, M.D. *Perfect Health: The Complete Mind/Body Guide.* New York: Harmony Books, 1991.

Colbin, Annemarie. *Food and Healing.* New York: Ballantine Books, 1996.

Frawley, David, OMD. *Ayurvedic Healing: A Comprehensive Guide.* Salt Lake City: Passage Press, 1989.

Lad, Usha and Dr. Vasant Lad. *Ayurvedic Cooking for Self-Healing.* Albuquerque: The Ayurvedic Press, 1997.

Lad, Vasant. *Ayurveda: The Science of Self-Healing*. Wilmot: Lotus Press, 1984.

Lad, Vasant. *The Complete Book of Ayurvedic Home Remedies*. New York: Harmony Books, 1998.

Morrison, Judith H. *The Ayurvedic Approach to Health and Longevity*. London: Gaia Books Ltd., 1995.

Pitchford, Paul. *Healing with Whole Foods: Oriental Traditions and Modern Nutrition*. Berkeley: North Atlantic Books, 1993.

Russell, David. "Self-Healing in Ayurvedic and Tibetan Medicines." Seminar: Kathmandu, Nepal. February 1994.

Shanbhag, Vivek, M.D. (Ayurveda), N.D. *A Beginner's Introduction to Ayurvedic Medicine*. New Canaan, Conn.: Keats Publishing, Inc., 1994.

Tiwari, Maya. *Ayurveda: A Life of Balance*. Rochester, N.Y.: Healing Arts Press, 1995.

Vernod, Dr. Virna. *Ayurveda for Life: Nutrition, Sexual Energy & Healing*. York Beach, Maine.: Samuel Weiser, Inc., 1997.

Chapter 7

Attwood, Charles, M.D., F.A.A.P. "Attention Deficit Disorder and Diet." *New Century Nutrition Archives*. http://www.newcenturynutrition.com/NCN/articles/attention.html (27 September 1999).

Balch, James F., M.D. and Phyllis A. Balch, C.N.C. *Prescription for Nutritional Healing*. New York: Avery Publishing Group, 1990.

Ballantine, Rudolph, M.D. *Radical Healing: Integrating the World's Great Therapeutic Traditions to Create a New Transformative Medicine.* New York: Harmony Books, 1999.

"BGH-Free Milk." *Genewatch.* February 1999. http://www.gene-watch.org/genewatch/genefeb.html (17 February 2000).

Boris, Marvin, M.D. and Francine S. Mandel, Ph.D. "Foods and Additives Are Common Causes of the Attention Deficit Hyperactive Disorder in Children." *Annals of Allergy* 72 (May 1994): 462–467.

Brewer, Susan M., Ph.D., R.D. and Patricia Kendall, Ph.D., R.D. "Position of the American Dietetic Association: Biotechnology and the Future of Food." 1996. http://www.eatright.org/abiotechnology.html (24 November 1999).

Brody, Jane E. "Diet Change May Avert Need for Ritalin." *New York Times,* November 2, 1999.

Brody, Jane E. *Jane Brody's Good Food Book.* New York: W. W. Norton & Co., 1985.

Campbell, Dr. T. Colin. "Do You Need Vitamin Supplements?" New Century Nutrition Archives. http://www.newcenturynutrition.com/NCN/ariticles/need_vitamins.html (27 September 1999).

Center for Science in the Public Interest. "America: Drowning in Sugar." August 3, 1999. http://www.cspinet/org/new/sugar.html (27 March 2000).

Center for Science in the Public Interest. "Scientists' Letters to the Department of Health and Human Services." October 25, 1999. http://www.cspinet.org/new/adhdletters.html (27 March 2000).

Center for Science in the Public Interest. "Stevia: Not Ready for Prime Time." March 21, 2000. http://www.cspinet.org/new/stevia.html (27 March 2000).

Center for Science in the Public Interest. "Studies Show That Diet May Trigger Adverse Behavior in Children." http://www.cspinet.org/new/adhdpr.html (27 March 2000).

Chubb, Lucy. "FDA Stonewalling on Sweetener, Activists Say." Environmental News Network. October 19, 1999. http://www.enn.com/news/enn-stories/1999/10/101999headache_6491.asp (11 March 2000).

Colbin, Annemarie. *Food and Healing*. New York: Ballantine Books, 1986.

Colbin, Annemarie. "Aspartame: The Real Story." 1997. http://www.foodandhealing.com/article-aspartame.htm (10 March 2000).

Consumers International. "Food Irradition: Solution or Threat?" June 29, 1999. http://193.128.6.150/consumers//campaigns/irradiation/irrad8.html (15 February 2000).

Council for Agricultural Science and Technology. "Radiation Pasteurization of Food." April 1996. http://www.cast-science.org/past_ip.htm (15 February 2000).

"A Cowboy in the Meat Business." *In Motion Magazine*. June 1997. http://www.purefood.org/coleman.html (19 September 1999).

Duffy, Valerie B., Ph.D., R.D. and G. Harvey Anderson, Ph.D. "Position of the American Dietetic Association: Use of Nutritive and Nonnutritive Sweeteners." *Journal of the American Dietetic Association* 98 (1998): 580–587.

Environmental Working Group. "What Pesticides Did You Eat Today?" http://www.foodnews.org/questions.html (13 March 2000).

Fukuoka, Masanobu. *The Natural Way of Farming: The Theory and Practice of Green Philosophy.* Tokyo: Japan Publications, 1985.

Gassen, Katzek, J., H.G. "Requirements of a System to Assess Possible Late Damage Caused by the Use of Genetic Engineering Methods in the Food Sector." *Ernahrungs-Umschau* 45, no. 1 (January 1998): 4.

Gibbs, Nancy. "The Age of Ritalin." *Time,* September 30, 1998.

Goldman, Larry, M.D., et al. "Diagnosis and Treatment of Attention-Deficit/Hyperactivity Disorder in Children and Adolescents." *Journal of the American Medical Association* 279, no. 14 (April 8, 1998): 1100–1106.

Hart, Kathleen. "Under Pressure American Medical Association Announces It Will Revise Its Policy on Safety of Genetically Engineered Foods." *Pesticide and Toxic Chemical News* 27, no. 45 (September 2, 1999). http://www.purefood.org/ge/amarevise.cfm (19 September 1999).

Hunt, Janet R., Ph.D., R.D. "Position of the American Dietetic Association: Vitamin and Mineral Supplementation." American Dietetic Association. http://www.eatright.org/asupple.html (24 November 1999).

Ivans, Molly. "Monsanto Displays a Record of Putting Technology Before Responsibility." *Arizona Daily Star.* January 9, 1999.

Jacobson, Michael F., Ph.D. and Bruce Maxwell. *What Are We Feeding Our Kids?* New York: Workman Publishing, 1994.

Johnson, Rachel K., Ph.D., M.P.H., R.D. and Theresa A. Nicklas, Dr.PH. "Position of the American Dietetic Association: Dietary Guidance for Healthy Children Aged 2 to 11 Years." *Journal of the American Dietetic Association* 99 (1999): 93–101.

Kennedy, Eileen, D.Sc., R.D. and Jeanne Goldberg, Ph.D., R.D. "What Are American Children Eating? Implications for Public Policy." *Nutrition Reviews* 53, no. 5 (May 1995): 111–126.

Kennedy, Rozella. "Genetically Engineered Foods: Too Many Unknowns; An Interview with John Fagan." *Mothering.* March/April 2000.

Knox, Jerry G., B.A., D.C. "Constipation." *Colon Therapy Journal.* August 1999.

Lilliston, Ben and Ronnie Cummins. "Organic Versus 'Organic': The Corruption of a Label." *The Ecologist.* July/August 1999. http://www.purfood.org/Organic/orgvsorg.htm (19 September 1999).

McCaleb, Rob. "Stevia Leaf—Too Good To Be Legal?" Herb Research Foundation. http://metalab.unc.edu/herbmed/mediher2.html (16 April 2000).

Mendieta, N. L. R., et al. "The Potential Allergenicity of Novel Foods." *Journal of the Science of Food and Agriculture* 75, no. 4 (December 1997): 405–411.

Ogden, Cynthia, Ph.D., et al. "Prevalence of Overweight Among Preschool Children in the United States, 1971 Through 1994." *Pediatrics* 99, no. 4 (1997): 593.

Olson, Robert E. "The Dietary Recommendations of the American Academy of Pediatrics." *American Journal of Clinical Nutrition* 61 (1995): 271–273.

Organic Consumers Association. "Food Irradiation Home Page." February 16, 2000. http://www.purefood.org/irradlink.html (17 February 2000).

Pitchford, Paul. *Healing with Whole Foods: Oriental Traditions and Modern Nutrition.* Berkeley: North Atlantic Books, 1993.

Rapp, Doris J., M.D. *Is This Your Child's World?* New York: Bantam Books, 1996.

Schardt, David. "Ritalin: Is It Safe?" *Nutrition Action Health Letter.* March 2000. http://www.cspinet.org/nah/3_00/diet_behavior.html (27 March 2000).

Sears, William, M.D. and Martha Sears, R.N. *The Family Nutrition Book: Everything You Need to Know About Feeding Your Children From Birth Through Adolescence.* New York: Little, Brown & Co., 1999.

Ticciati, Laura and Robin Ticciati, Ph.D. *Genetically Engineered Foods: Are They Safe? You Decide.* Los Angeles: Keats Publishing, 1998.

Weil, Andrew, M.D. *Eating Well for Optimum Health: The Essential Guide to Food, Diet, and Nutrition.* New York: Alfred A. Knopf, 2000.

Wood, Olivia Bennett, M.P.H., R.D. and Christine M. Bruhn, Ph.D. "Position of the American Dietetic Association: Food Irradiation." 1995. http://www.eatright.org/airradi.html (15 February 2000).

Chapter 8

Bell, Iris R., M.D., Ph.D., F.A.C.N., et al. "Symptom and Personality Profiles of Young Adults from a College Student Population with Self-Reported Illness from Foods and Chemicals." *Journal of the American College of Nutrition* 12, no. 6 (1993): 693–702.

Bell, Iris R., M.D., Ph.D., et al. "Psychological Characteristics and Subjective Intolerance for Xenobiotic Agents of Normal Young Adults with Trait Shyness and Defensiveness." *Journal of Nervous and Mental Disease* 182, no. 7 (July 1994): 367–374.

Bell, Iris R., M.D., Ph.D., et al. "Individual Differences in Neural Sensitization and the Role of Context in Illness from Low-Level Environmental Chemical Exposures." *Environmental Health Perspectives* 105, Supplement 2 (March 1997): 457–466.

Berkson, Jacob B. *A Canary's Tale.* Jacob B. Berkson, 1997.

Berthold-Bond, Annie. *Better Basics for the Home: Simple Solutions for Less Toxic Living.* New York: Three Rivers Press, 1999.

Burros, Marian. "Plastic Wrap Worries Rise Amid New Studies." *Milwaukee Journal Sentinel,* March 3, 1999.

California Medical Association Scientific Board Task Force on Clinical Ecology. "Clinical Ecology—A Critical Appraisal." *Western Journal of Medicine* 144 (February 1986): 239–245.

Carson, Rachel. *Silent Spring.* Boston, Mass.: Houghton Mifflin, 1962.

Colburn, Theo, Dianne Dumanoski, and John Peterson Myers. *Our Stolen Future: Are We Threatening Our Fertility, Intelligence, and Survival?* New York: Dutton, 1996.

Dadd, Debra Lynn. *Nontoxic, Natural & Earthwise.* Los Angeles: Jeremy P. Tarcher, Inc., 1990.

Environmental Protection Agency. "The Inside Story—A Guide to Indoor Air Quality." http://www.epa.gov/iaq/pubs/insidest.html (1 February 2000).

Geissinger, Steve. "Report: Use of Pesticides Up." *San Francisco Chronicle,* May 4, 2000.

Kahn, Ephraim, M.D., M.P.H. and Gideon Letz, M.D., M.P.H. "Clinical Ecology: Environmental Medicine or Unsubstantiated Theory?" *Annals of Internal Medicine* 111, no. 2 (15 July 1989): 104–105.

Kellas, William Randall, Ph.D. and Andrea Sharon Dworkin, Ph.D. *Surviving the Toxic Crisis.* Olivenhaven, CA: Professional Preference, 1996.

Kellas, William Randall, Ph.D. and Andrea Sharon Dworkin, Ph.D. *Thriving in a Toxic World.* Olivenhaven, CA: Professional Preference, 1996.

Pennybacker, Mindy, ed. *The Green Guide Newsletters,* Nos. 20–75. New York: Mothers & Others for a Livable Planet, Inc., 1996–2000.

Pennybacker, Mindy and Aisha Ikramuddin. *Mothers & Others for a Livable Planet's Guide to Natural Baby Care.* New York: John Wiley & Sons, Inc., 1999.

Radetsky, Peter. *Allergic to the 20th Century.* Boston: Little, Brown and Company, 1997.

Rapp, Doris J., M.D. *Is This Your Child's World?* New York: Bantam Books, 1996.

Terr, Abba I., M.D. "Environmental Illness: A Clinical Review of 50 Cases." *Archives of Internal Medicine* 146 (January 1986): 145–149.

Chapter 9

Altemeier, William A., M.D. "Take Your Tricks Where You See Them." *Pediatric Annals* 26, no. 6 (June 1997): 345–351.

American Academy of Pediatrics, Committee on Infectious Diseases. "Measles: Reassessment of the Current Immunization Policy." *Pediatrics* 84, no. 6 (December 1989): 1110–1113.

Arbeter, Allan M., M.D., et al. "Varicella Vaccine Studies in Healthy Children and Adults." *Pediatrics* 78 (Supplement 1986): 748–756.

Arvin, Ann M., M.D. "Live Attenuated Varicella Vaccine." *Pediatric Annals* no. 6 (June 1997): 384–388.

Bloch, Alan B., M.D., et al. "Health Impact of Measles Vaccination in the United States." *Pediatrics* 76, no. 4 (October 1985): 524–532.

Buttram, Harold, M.D. and John Chriss Hoffman, Ph.D. *Vaccinations and Immune Malfunction.* Richlandtown, Pa.: The Humanitarian Publishing Company, 1995.

Centers for Disease Control and Prevention. "Healthy People 2000." http://www.cdc.gov/ncidod/healthypeople/2000/idachievechall.htm. (15 May 2000)

Chaitow, Leon. *Vaccinations and Immunizations: Dangers, Delusions, and Alternatives.* London, England: C. W. Daniel Company Ltd., 1990.

Coulter, Harris L. and Barbara Loe Fisher. *A Shot in the Dark.* Garden City Park, N.Y.: Avery Publishing Group, 1991.

Evans, Geoffrey, M.D. "National Childhood Vaccine Injury Act: Revision of the Vaccine Injury Table." *Pediatrics* 998, no. 6 (December 1996): 1179–1181.

Fisher, Barbara Loe. *The Consumer's Guide to Childhood Vaccines.* Vienna: National Vaccine Information Center, 1997.

Guris, Dalya, M.D., M.P.H., et al. "Pertussis Vaccination in the United States—New Developments and Recommendations." *Pediatric Annals* 26, no. 6 (June 1997): 374.

Hull, Harry F., M.D., et al. "Risk Factors for Measles Vaccine Failure Among Immunized Students." *Pediatrics* 76, no. 4 (October 1985): 518–523.

James, Walene. *Immunization: The Reality Behind the Myth.* Westport: Bergin & Garvey, 1995.

Kimberlin, David W., M.D. "Rubella Immunization." *Pediatric Annals* 26, no. 6 (June 1997): 366–370.

Lieu, Tracy A., M.D., M.P.H., et al. "Would Better Adherence to Guidelines Improve Childhood Immunization Rates?" *Pediatrics* 98, no. 6 (December 1996): 1062–1068.

MacNalty, Sir Arthur Salusbury, K.C.B. "The Prevention of Smallpox: From Edward Jenner to Mockton Copeman." *British Medical Journal* 2 vol. 519, no. 946 (1966) 1–14.

Mendelsohn, Robert S., M.D. *How to Raise a Healthy Child. . . in Spite of Your Doctor.* New York: Ballantine Books, 1984.

Miller, Neil Z. *Immunization: Theory vs. Reality.* Santa Fe: New Atlantean Press, 1996.

Miller, Neil Z. "Vaccines and Natural Health." *Mothering,* Spring 1994: 44–54.

Miller, Neil Z. *Vaccines: Are They Really Safe and Effective?* Santa Fe: New Atlantean Press, 1994.

Morbidity and Mortality Weekly Report (MMWR) 45, no. RR-12 (September 6, 1996): 2.

Morbidity and Mortality Weekly Report (MMWR) 46, no. 35 (September 5, 1997): 822–826.

Murphy, James. *What Every Parent Should Know About Childhood Immunization.* Dennis, Mass.: Earth Healing Products, 1993.

Neustaedter, Randall, O.M.D., L.ac. *The Immunization Decision.* Berkeley: North Atlantic Books, 1990.

Neustaedter, Randall, O.M.D., L.ac. *The Vaccine Guide.* Berkeley: North Atlantic Books, 1996.

Offit, Paul A. and Louis M. Bell. *What Every Parent Should Know About Vaccines.* New York: Macmillan, 1998.

O'Mara, Peggy, ed. "Vaccination: The Issue of Our Times." *Mothering Magazine* (1997).

O'Mara, Peggy, ed. "Vaccinations: The Rest of the Story; A Selection of Articles, Letters, and Resources 1979–1992." *Mothering Magazine* (1992).

Plotkin, Stanley, M.D. and Edward Mortimer, M.D., eds. *Vaccines,* 2d ed. Philadelphia: W. B. Saunders Co., 1994.

Preblud, Stephen R., M.D. "Varicella: Complications and Cost." *Pediatrics* 78 (Supplement 1986): 728–735.

"Review of the First International Public Conference on Vaccination," *Mothering Magazine,* no. 86 (Jan./Feb. 1998).

Rozario, Diane. *The Immunization Resource Guide.* Burlington, Iowa: Patter Publications, 1995.

Scheibner, Viera, Ph.D. *Vaccination: The Medical Assault on the Immune System.* Blackheath, NSW, Australia: V. Scheibner, 1993.

Schrof, Joannie M. "Miracle Vaccines." *U.S. News & World Report.* November 23, 1998.

Severyn, Kristine M., R.Ph., Ph.D. *Vaccine News.* Issues 1995–2000.

Shepherd, Dorothy, M.D. *Homeopathy in Epidemic Diseases.* Rustington, Essex, U.K.: Health Sciences Press, 1967.

Tanouye, Elysee. "The Vaccine Business Gets a Shot in the Arm." *Wall Street Journal,* February 25, 1998.

"Vaccination: The Issue of Our Times." *Mothering,* Summer 1996.

Waisbren, Burton A., Sr., M.D. "The Hepatitis B Vaccination Debate: Should Children Be Universally Vaccinated?" *Medical Crossfire,* March 2000. http://wwwm.medical crossfire.com/debate_archive/March_oo/HepatitisB.htm (8 May 2000).

Chapter 10

American Dental Association. "Dental Materials." 1999. http://www.ada.org/consumer/faq/dent-mat.html.

American Dental Association. "Fluoridation Facts." 1999. http://www.ada.org/consumer/fluoride/facts/benefits.html.

American Dental Association News Releases. "Dental Amalgam: 150 Years of Safety and Effectiveness." 1995. http://www.ada.org/newsrel/1195/nr-02a.html.

American Dental Association News Releases. "International Experts Report: No Amalgam Bans in Effect." 1996. http://www.ada.org/newsrel/9612/nr-03.html.

American Dietetic Association. "Position of the American Dietetic Association: The Impact of Fluoride on Dental Health." *Journal of the American Dietetic Association* 94 (1994). http://www.eatright.org/fluoride.html (24 November 1999).

"Biological and Mercury Free Dentistry." 1999. http://www.medical-library.net/specialties/_biological_and_mercury_free_dentistry.html (17 December 1999).

Breiner, Mark A., D.D.S. *Whole-Body Dentistry*. Fairfield: Quantum Health Press, 1999.

Canedy, Dana. "Toothpaste a Hazard? Just Ask the F.D.A." *New York Times,* March 24, 1998.

Colquhoun, John. "Why I Changed My Mind About Water Fluoridation." *Perspectives in Biology and Medicine* 41, no. 1, Autumn 1997. http://www.cadvision.com/fluoride/colquh.htm (6 December 1999).

The Doctor's Medical Library. "Biological and Mercury Free Dentistry." http://www.medical-library.net/specialties/_biological_and_mercury_free_dentistry.html (17 December 1999).

Downey, Michael. "A Crack Appears in the Fluoride Front." *Toronto Star,* April 25, 1999.

Duerksen, Susan. "The Fluoride Debate." *San Diego Union-Tribune,* September 1, 1999.

Duerksen, Susan. "Staining of Teeth on Increase in Treated, Nontreated Areas." *San Diego Union-Tribune,* September 1, 1999.

Easley, Dr. Michael W. "Fluoridation: A Triumph of Science over Propaganda." American Council on Science and Health. 1997 and 1998. http://www.acsh.org/publications/priorities/0804/fluoridation.html (6 December 1999).

Eley, B. M. "The Future of Dental Amalgam: A Review of the Literature." *British Dental Journal* 182, no. 12 (June 28, 1997): 455–459.

"Fluoride May Be Linked to Brain Tissue Damage." *Medical Industry Today,* April 20, 1998.

Gerber, Richard, M.D. *Vibrational Medicine: New Choices for Healing Ourselves.* Santa Fe: Bear & Company, 1988.

Halbach, S., et al. "Systemic Transfer of Mercury from Amalgam Fillings Before and After Cessation of Emission." *Environ Res* 77, no. 2 (May 1998): 115–23.

Hardy, Dr. James E. *Mercury-Free: The Wisdom Behind the Global Consumer Movement to Ban "Silver" Dental Fillings.* Glassboro, N.J.: Gabriel Rose Press, Inc., 1996.

"Heed Fluoride Warnings." *Tampa Tribune,* November 19, 1999.

Hill, David R. "Fluoride: Risks and Benefits?" August 1997. http://www.cadvision.com/fluoride/calgaryh.htm (6 December 1999).

Huggins, Hal A., D.D.S., M.S. *It's All in Your Head: The Link Between Mercury Amalgams and Illness*. Garden City Park, N.Y.: Avery Publishing Group, Inc., 1993.

Huggins, Hal A., D.D.S., M.S. *Uninformed Consent: The Hidden Dangers in Dental Care*. Charlottesville, VA: Hampton Roads Publishing, Co., 1999.

James, George. "Fluoride, A Missing Ingredient." *New York Times*, April 18, 1999.

Jerome, Frank J., D.D.S. *Tooth Truth: A Patient's Guide to Metal-Free Dentistry*. San Diego: ProMotion Publishing, 1995.

Jones, D. W. "Exposure or Absorption and the Crucial Questions of Limits for Mercury." *Journal of the Canadian Dental Association* 65, no. 1 (January 1999): 42–46.

Kennedy, David, D.D.S. *How to Save Your Teeth: Toxic-Free Preventive Dentistry*. Delaware, Ohio: Health Action Press, 1996.

Oskarsson, A., et al. "Total and Inorganic Mercury in Breast Milk in Relation to Fish Consumption and Amalgam in Lactating Women." *Archives of Environmental Health* 51, no. 3 (May–June 1996): 234–41.

Parker-Pope, Tara. "Some Young Children Get Too Much Fluoride in Caring for Teeth." *Wall Street Journal*, December 21, 1998.

Pleva, J. "Dental Mercury—A Public Health Hazard." *Review of Environmental Health* 10, no. 1 (Jan.–March 1994): 1–27.

Ring, Marvin E., D.D.S. *Dentistry: An Illustrated History*. New York: Abrams, 1985.

Royal, Michael A. "Amalgam Fillings: Do Dental Patients Have a Right to Informed Consent?" http://www.fplc.edu/risk/vol2/spring/royal.htm (3 December 1999).

Sherrell, Darlene. "What's Wrong with Fluoridation? Follow the Money." http://www.rvi.net/^fluoride/wrong.htm (13 December 99).

Snapp, K. R., et al. "The Contribution of Dental Amalgam to Mercury in Blood." *Journal of Dental Restoration* 68, no. 5 (May 1968): 780–785.

"Summary of Key Studies." http://www.nofluoride.com/summary.htm (13 December 99).

Timmons, Eamon. "Fluoride Causes Disease, Doctor Claims." *Irish Times,* August 16, 1999.

Weiner, J. A. and M. Nylander. "An Estimation of the Uptake of Mercury from Amalgam Fillings Based on Urinary Excretion of Mercury in Swedish Subjects." *Science of the Total Environment* 168, no. 3 (June 30, 1995): 255–265.

Weiner, J. A., et al. "Does Mercury from Amalgam Restorations Constitute a Health Hazard?" *Science of the Total Environment* 99, no. 1–2 (December 1990): 1–22.

Yiamouyiannis, John, Ph.D. *Fluoride the Aging Factor: How to Recognize and Avoid the Devastating Effects of Fluoride.* Delaware, OH: Health Action Press, 1986.

Ziff, Sam and Michael F. Ziff, D.D.S. *Dentistry Without Mercury.* Orlando: Bio-Probe, Inc., 1995.

Ziff, Sam and Michael F. Ziff, D.D.S. *Infertility & Birth Defects.* Orlando: Bio-Probe, Inc., 1987.

Chapter 11

"Acupuncture Laws by State." http://www.acupuncture.com/StateLaws/StateLaws.htm (29 January 2000).

Andrews, Michelle. "The Doctor Will See Your Soul Now." *Smart Money,* December 1999.

Angell, Marcia, M.D. and Jerome P. Kassirer, M.D. "Alternative Medicine—The Risks of Untested and Unregulated Remedies." *New England Journal of Medicine* 339, no. 12 (September 17, 1998): 839–841.

Barrett, Stephen and William T. Jarvis. *The Health Robbers: A Close Look at Quackery in America.* Buffalo: Prometheus Books, 1993.

Beyerstein, Barry. "Social and Judgmental Biases That Make Inert Treatments Seem to Work." *Scientific Review of Alternative Medicine* 3, no.2 (1999): 20–33.

Butler, Kurt. *The Consumer's Guide to Alternative Medicine: A Close Look at Homeopathy, Acupuncture, Faith-Healing, and Other Unconventional Treatments.* Buffalo: Prometheus Books, 1992.

Fauber, John. "Activist Assails Modern Quackery." *Milwaukee Journal Sentinel,* March 31, 1997.

Fishbein, Morris, M.D. *The History of the American Medical Association 1847 to 1947.* Philadelphia: W. B. Saunders & Co., 1947.

Gordon, Hunter R. "A Review of the SRAM Conference in Philadelphia." *The Scientific Review of Alternative Medicine.* http://www.hcrc.org/sram/conf-rep.html (23 January 2000).

Harman, William. "What Are Noetic Sciences?" *Noetic Sciences Review* 47 (Winter 1998): 32–33.

"Institute of Noetic Sciences Programs of Research." *Institute of Noetic Sciences.* http://www.noetic.org/Ions/research/program_modules.asp (24 January 2000).

Jakleui, Mary Chris. "Physician Compensation Growth Slows." *Modern Healthcare,* August 2, 1999.

Jaroff, Leon. "Government Has No Business Legitimizing Quackery." *Houston Chronicle.* October 7, 1997.

Kolata, Gina and Kurt Eichenwald. "Health Business Thrives on Unproven Treatment, Leaving Science Behind." *New York Times on the Web,* October 3, 1999. http://www.nytimes.com/library/national/science/health/100399cancer-test.html (3 October 1999).

Lewis, Shawn D. "Dose of Caution: Beware of Quacks in Alternative Medicine." *The Detroit News,* February 2, 1996.

National Council Against Health Fraud. "Position Paper on Homeopathy." http://www.hcrc.org/ncahf/pos-pap/homeop.html (9 January 2000).

Perlman, David. "New Medical Journal Offers Alternatives." *Houston Chronicle,* January 11, 1998.

"Quotations by Galileo Galilei." http://www-groups.dcs.st-and.ac.uk/~history/Quotations/Galileo.html (18 January 2000).

Relman, Arnold S. "A Trip to Stonesville." *New Republic,* December 14, 1998.

Russek, Linda G., Ph.D. and Gary E. Schwartz, Ph.D. "Interpersonal Heart-Brain Registration and the Perception of Parental Love: A 42-Year Follow-Up of the Harvard Mastery of Stress Study." *Subtle Energies* 5, no. 3 (1994): 195–208.

Schissel, Marvin J., D.D.S. and John E. Dodes, D.D.S. *The Whole Tooth: How to Find a Good Dentist, Keep Healthy Teeth, and Avoid the Incompetents, Quacks, and Frauds.* New York: St. Martin's Press, 1997.

Schwartz, Gary, Ph.D., et al. "Electrostatic Body-Motion Registration and the Human Antenna-Receiver Effect: A New Method for Investigating Interpersonal Dynamical Energy System Interactions." *Subtle Energies & Energy Medicine* 7, no. 2: 149–184.

"A Statement in Defense of Scientific Medicine from the Council for Scientific Medicine." *Scientific Review of Alternative Medicine.* http://hcrc.org/sram/defense.html (23 January 2000).

Chapter 12

American Academy of Pediatrics. "Policy Statement: Children, Adolescents, and Television." *Pediatrics* 96, no. 4 (October 1995): 786–787.

Aronson, Linda Crispell. *Big Spirits, Little Bodies: Parenting Your Way to Wholeness.* Virginia Beach: A.R.E. Press, 1995.

Catalfo, Phil. *Raising Spiritual Children in a Material World: Introducing Spirituality into Family Life.* New York: Berkley Books, 1997.

Cohen, Marion. "Rethinking Creativity." *Mothering,* no. 71 (Summer 1994): 63–67.

Doe, Mimi and Marsha Walch, Ph.D. *10 Principles for Spiritual Parenting: Nurturing Your Child's Soul.* New York: HarperCollins, 1998.

Dossey, Larry, M.D. "Creativity: On Intelligence, Insight, and the Cosmic Soup." *Alternative Therapies in Health and Medicine* 6, no. 1 (January 2000): 12–18.

Glazer, Steven, ed. *The Heart of Learning; Spirituality in Education.* New York: Jeremy P. Tarcher, 1999.

Healy, Jane M. "Understanding TV's Effects on the Developing Brain." *American Academy of Pediatrics News,* May 1998. http://www.aap.org/advocacy/chm98nws.htm (21 March 2000).

Kabat-Zinn, Mayla and Jon Kabat-Zinn. *Everyday Blessings: The Inner Work of Mindful Parenting.* New York: Hyperion, 1997.

Kondracke, Morton. "Don't Kill Your TV to Reduce Total Viewing Hours, Just Bind and Gag It." *Arizona Daily Star,* August 30, 1997.

Lewis, Richard. *Living By Wonder: The Imaginative Life of Childhood.* New York: Parabola Books, 1998.

Moore, Thomas. *Care of the Soul.* New York: HarperPerennial, 1994.

Oppenheimer, Todd. "Schooling the Imagination." *Atlantic Monthly,* September, 1999.

Rich, Michael, M.D., M.P.H., F.A.A.P. "Pediatricians Should Educate Parents, Youths About Media's Effects." *American Academy of Pediatric News,* September 1999. http://www.aap.org./advocacy/rich999.htm (21 March 2000).

Shifrin, Donald, M.D., F.A.A.P. "Three-Year Study Documents Nature of Television Violence." *American Academy of Pediatric News,* August 1998. http://www.aap.org. advocacy/shifrin898.htm (21 March 2000).

Signorielli, Nancy, Ph.D. "Television and the Perpetuation of Gender-Role Stereotypes." *American Academy of Pediatric News,* February 1998. http://www.aap.org./advocacy/ sign298.htm (21 March 2000).

Spangler, David. *Parent as Mystic, Mystic as Parent.* New York: Riverhead Books, 1998.

TV Turnoff Network. "Our Television Habit." http://www.tvturnoff.org/FactsandfigPage.htm (19 May 2000).

RESOURCES

Ayurveda

American Institute of Vedic Studies
P.O. Box 8357
Santa Fe, NM 87504-8357
Telephone: (505) 983-9385
Fax: (505) 982-5807
E-mail: vedanet@aol.com
Web site: www.vedanet.com

Dr. David Frawley's institution. Web site includes course work info, books, articles, and summary of doshas.

The Ayurvedic Institute
11311 Menaul NE
Albuquerque, NM 87112
Telephone: (505) 291-9698
Fax: (505) 294-7572
E-mail: info@ayurveda.com (for questions on products only)
Web site: www.ayurveda.com

One of the leading Ayurveda schools outside of India. Created and directed by Dr. Vasant Lad. Check out Web site for books, herbs, and Ayurvedic therapies.

Maharishi Ayurveda Products
1068 Elkton Drive
Colorado Springs, Co 80907
Telephone: 800-255-8322 or (719) 260-7400
Fax: (719) 260-7400
E-mail: info@mapi.com (for questions on products only)
Web site: www.mapi.com

Web site provides information on products, herbs, recipes, and published research. Newsletter also available on-line that views critical health issues from the perspective of Maharishi Ayurveda.

Herbal Medicine

The American Botanical Council
6200 Manor Road
Austin, TX 78723
or
P.O. Box 144345
Austin, TX 78714-4345
Telephone: (512) 926-4900
Fax: (512) 926-2345
E-mail: abc@herbalgram.org
Web site: www.herbalgram.org

The leading nonprofit educational and research organization disseminating science-based information that promotes the safe and effective use of medicinal plants and phytomedicines. To request a free Herbal Education Catalog, call 1-800-373-7105.

The American Herbalists Guild
P.O. Box 70
Roosevelt, UT 84066
Telephone: (435) 722-8434
Fax: (435) 722-8452
E-mail: ahgoffice@earthlink.net
Web site: www.healthy.net/herbalists/

A nonprofit membership-based organization representing the goals and voices of herbalists interested in promoting standards of excellence in education, ethics, and professional competency. AHG is the only professional, peer-reviewed organization in the United States for clinical and traditional herbalists.

Herb Research Foundation
1007 Pearl Street, #200
Boulder, CO 80302
Telephone: (303) 449-2265
Fax: (303) 449-7849
Web site: www.herbs.org

A nonprofit membership-based organization providing current research on herbs. Publishes HerbalGram and Herbs for Health. Web site: http://planetherbs.com

Dr. Michael Tierra, L.Ac., O.M.D.
Web site: http://planetherbs.com

Author of Planetary Herbology and Way of Herbs. Dr. Tierra's comprehensive Web site covers such topics as how to assemble an herbal first aid kit, the history of herbal medicine, and Chinese, Ayurvedic, and Western herbal medicines.

Holistic Dentistry

Bio-Probe, Inc.
P.O. Box 608010
Orlando, FL 32860-8010
Telephone: (407) 290-9670
Fax: (407) 299-4149
E-mail: hgsz@aol.com
Web site: www.bioprobe.com

Sells books on dental issues, especially those relating to amalgam. Also carries specialized products for dentists working mercury free. (For referrals to mercury-free dentists contact the International Academy of Oral Medicine and Toxicology, listed below.)

Citizens for Safe Drinking Water
1010 University Avenue, #52
San Diego, CA 92103
Telephone: 1-800-728-3833
Fax: (619) 281-1578
E-mail: greenjeff@home.com
Provides scientific materials and data about fluoride to organizations and individuals. Goal is to assure that individuals making decisions concerning fluoridation of public drinking water are well informed.

International Academy of Oral Medicine and Toxicology (IAOMT)
P.O. Box 608531
Orlando, FL 32860
Telephone: (407) 298-2450
Fax: (407) 298-3075
E-mail: mziff@iaomt.org
Web site: www.iaomt.org
Membership-based organization composed of mercury-free dentists, physicians, and research scientists interested in biocompatibility of dental materials. Provides referrals to mercury-free dentists nationwide. Membership not required for this free service.

Homeopathy

Homeopathic Educational Services
2036 Blake Street
Berkeley, CA 94704
Telephone: (510) 649-0294
Fax:(510) 649-1955
E-mail: mail@homeopathic.com
Web site: www.homeopathic.com

Leading resource center for homeopathic books, tapes, medicine kits, software, and distance learning programs. Web site posts 100 free articles on homeopathy, as well as an on-line catalog, and includes information on remedies for children and infants and how to locate a homeopath in your area.

National Center for Homeopathy
801 North Fairfax, #306
Alexandria, VA 22314
Telephone: (703) 548-7790
Fax: (703) 548-7792
E-mail: info@homeopathic.org
Web site: www.homeopathic.org

Promotes homeopathy to general public and professional homeopaths. Provides educational material and resources. Web site includes information on finding a homeopath.

Immunizations

The Immunization Resource Guide: Where to Find Answers to All Your Questions About Childhood Immunizations
by Diane Rozario
Patter Publications
P.O. Box 204
Burlington, IA 52601

Everyone who faces the vaccine decision needs a copy of this invaluable resource guide, which reviews over 85 books covering all aspects of childhood vaccinations and and lists over 130 vaccine organizations and resources. Order directly from Patter Publications. The cost is $13.95.

National Vaccine Information Center (NVIC)
512 W. Maple Avenue, Suite 206
Vienna, VA 22180
Telephone: 1-800-909-SHOT or (703) 938-DPT3
Fax: (703) 938-5768
E-mail:info@909shot.com
Web site: www.909shot.com

A nonprofit educational organization dedicated to the prevention of vaccine injuries and deaths through public education. Assists parents of vaccine-damaged children, promotes research to evaluate vaccine safety and effectiveness, and monitors vaccine research, development, policy making, and legislation.

Vaccine Policy Institute
251 W. Ridgeway Drive
Dayton, OH 45459
Telephone: (937) 435-4750
Fax: (937) 435-4750

Kristine M. Severyn, R.Ph., Ph.D., directs this nonprofit organization and writes the newsletter Vaccine News. *Loaded with scientific information about vaccines, this newsletter is a must-read for laypeople and professionals. Call to order.*

Vaccine Exemptions:
Special Human Rights Services
Grace Girdwain
8320 S. Nashville Avenue
Burbank, IL 60459-2333

To Report an Adverse Vaccine Reaction:
Vaccine Adverse Event Reporting System (VAERS)
Telephone: 1-800-822-7967

To File a Claim for a Vaccine Injury:
National Vaccine Injury Compensation Program of the
U.S. Public Health Service
Telephone: 1-800-338-2382

Nutrition and the Environment

Aspartame Consumer Safety Network
P.O. Box 780634
Dallas, TX 75378
Telephone: (214) 352-4268
E-Mail: marystod@airmail.net
Web site: http://web2.airmail.net/marystod
Consumer advocacy group providing education about aspartame.

Center for Science in the Public Interest
1875 Connecticut Avenue, NW
Suite 300
Washington, D.C. 20009
Telephone: (202) 332-9110
Fax: (202) 265-4954
E-mail: cspi@cspinet.org
Web site: http://www.cspinet.com
A nonprofit education and advocacy organization that strives to educate the public about nutrition and alcohol. Works to improve the safety of our food supply. Publishes the Nutrition Action Healthletter.

Environmental Working Group
1718 Connecticut Avenue, N.W.
Suite 600
Washington, D.C. 20009
Telephone: (202) 667-6982
Fax (202) 232-2592
E-mail: info@ewg.org
Web site: http://www.ewg.org

To find out if your child's diet exceeds the government safety stan-dards for pesticides that harm the nervous system, go to this site's "FoodNews.org" section and click on "Kids' Corner."

Mothers & Others for a Liveable Planet
40 W. 20th Street
New York, NY 10011-4211
Telephone: 1-888-ECO-INFO
Fax: (212) 242-1545
E-mail: mothers@mothers.org
Web site: http://www.mothers.org

Excellent resource for environmental and nutritional topics. Started with the help of Meryl Streep. Publishes the Green Guide monthly newsletter, which is chock full of scientific information about topics like organic food, genetically engineered food, and pesticides. A very practical resource.

Organic Consumers Association
6114 Highway 61
Little Marais, MN 55614
Telephone: (218) 226-4164
Fax: (218) 226-4157
E-mail: alliance@mr.net
Web site: http://www.purefood.org

Promotes food safety, organic farming, and sustainable agriculture practices in the United States and internationally. Web site pro-vides articles on genetic engineering, food irradiation, toxic sludge fertilizer, mad cow disease, and rBGH.

Pesticide Action Network North America (PANNA)
49 Powell Street, Suite 500
San Francisco, CA 94102
Telephone: (415) 981-1771
Fax: (415) 981-1991
E-mail: panna@panna.org
Web site: http://www.panna.org

PANNA is a nonprofit organization working to advance sustainable alternatives to pesticides worldwide. To subscribe to its weekly e-mail news service—Pesticide Action Network Updates Service (PANUPS), which provides resource guides and reports on pesticide issues not always covered by the mainstream media—send a blank e-mail message to panups-subscribe@igc.topica.com.

Practical Allergy Research Foundation (P.A.R.F.)
P.O. Box 60
Buffalo, NY 14223-0060
Telephone: (716) 875-0398
Fax: (716) 875-5399
Web site: http://www.drrzpp.com

Educates parents about allergies and chemical sensitivities and provides solutions for living with these conditions in home and school environments. Books, audio tapes, and video tapes are available.

Other Publications

Healthy Child
Future Generations
1275 Fourth Street, Suite 118
Santa Rosa, CA 95404
E-mail: editor@healthychild.com
Web site: http://www.healthychild.com

A newsletter about raising healthy children. Well-researched articles on topics including nutrition, immunizations, pesticides, fluoride, and herbal medicine. Web site also posts articles and is definitely worth a look.

Real Life
245 Eighth Avenue
PMB 400
New York, NY 10011
Telephone: (802) 893-7040 (phone line at Fairfax, Vermont, office)

Gem of a magazine, much of it written in a warm tone with gentle humor. Informative articles cover the environment, nutrition, stress-reducers for parents, and exercise. Includes parenting and other inspirational essays. Call to receive a trial issue.

RECOMMENDED READING

Balch, James F., M.D. and Phyllis A. Balch, C.N.C. *Prescription for Nutritional Healing: A Practical A–Z Reference to Drug-Free Remedies Using Vitamins, Minerals, Herbs & Food Supplements.* Garden City Park, NY: Avery Publishing Group, Inc.

Ballentine, Rudolph, M.D. *Radical Healing: Integrating the World's Great Therapeutic Traditions to Create a New Transformative Medicine.* New York: Harmony Books, 1999.

Beinfield, Harriet, L.Ac. and Efrem Korngold, L.Ac., O.M.D. *Between Heaven and Earth: A Guide to Chinese Medicine.* New York: Ballantine Books, 1991.

Berthold-Bond, Annie. *Better Basics for the Home: Simple Solutions for Less Toxic Living.* New York: Three Rivers Press, 1999.

Capra, Fritjof. *The Turning Point: Science, Society, and the Rising Culture.* New York: Bantam Books, 1982.

Colbin, Annemarie. *Food and Healing.* New York: Ballantine Books, 1996.

Coulter, Harris L. and Barbara Loe Fisher. *A Shot in the Dark: Why the P in the DPT Vaccination May Be Hazardous to Your Child's Health.* Garden City Park, NY: Avery Publishing Group, Inc., 1991.

Dodt, Colleen K. *Natural BabyCare: Pure and Soothing Recipes and Techniques for Mothers and Babies.* Pownal, VT: Storey Books, 1997.

Gladstar, Rosemary. *Herbal Remedies for Children's Health.* Pownal, VT: Storey Books, 1999.

Hardy, James E., D.D.S. *Mercury Free: The Wisdom Behind the Global Consumer Movement to Ban "Silver" Dental Fillings.* Glassboro, NJ: Gabriel Rose Press, Inc., 1996.

Kabat-Zinn, Myla and Jon Kabat-Zinn. *Everyday Blessings: The Inner Work of Mindful Parenting.* New York: Hyperion, 1997.

Kennedy, David, D.D.S. *How to Save Your Teeth: Toxic-Free Preventive Dentistry.* Delaware, OH: Health Action Press, 1993.

Kunz, Dora, ed. *Spiritual Healing: Doctors Examine Therapeutic Touch and Other Holistic Treatments.* Wheaton: The Theosophical Publishing House, 1985.

Lad, Vasant. *The Complete Book of Ayurvedic Home Remedies.* New York: Harmony Books, 1998.

Lewis, Richard. *Living by Wonder: Writings on the Imaginative Life of Childhood.* New York: Parabola Books, 1998.

Morningstar, Amadea with Urmila Desai. *The Ayurvedic Cookbook.* Wilmot, WI: Lotus Press, 1990.

Morrison, Judith H. *The Book of Ayurveda: A Holistic Approach to Health and Longevity.* London: Gaia Books Limited, 1995.

Neustaedter, Randall, O.M.D. *The Vaccine Guide: Making an Informed Choice.* Berkeley: North Atlantic Books, 1996.

Ody, Penelope. *Home Herbal: A Practical Guide to Making Herbal Remedies for Common Ailments.* New York: DK Publishing, Inc., 1995.

O'Mara, Peggy with Jane McConnell. *Natural Family Living: The Mothering Magazine Guide to Parenting.* New York: Pocket Books, 2000.

Pennybacker, Mindy and Aisha Ikramuddin. *Mothers & Others for a Liveable Planet Guide to Natural Baby Care.* New York: John Wiley & Sons, Inc., 1999.

Pitchford, Paul. *Healing with Whole Foods: Oriental Traditions and Modern Nutrition.* Berkeley: North Atlantic Books, 1993.

Rapp, Doris J., M.D. *Is This Your Child's World? How You Can Fix the Schools and Homes That Are Making Your Children Sick.* New York: Bantam Books, 1996.

Reder, Alan, Phil Catalfo, and Stephanie Renfrow. *The Whole Parenting Guide: Strategies, Resources, and Inspiring Stories for Holistic Parenting and Family Living.* New York: Broadway Books, 1999.

Scheibner, Viera, Ph.D. *Vaccination: The Medical Assault on the Immune System.* Blackheath, NSW, Australia: V. Scheibner, 1993.

Scott, Julian, Ph.D. *Natural Medicine for Children: Drug-Free Health Care for Children from Birth to Age Twelve.* London: Gaia Books Limited, 1990.

Sears, William, M.D. and Martha Sears, R.N. *The Family Nutrition Book: Everything You Need to Know About Feeding Your Children from Birth Through Adolescence.* New York: Little, Brown & Co., 1999.

Shepherd, Dorothy, M.D. *Homeopathy in Epidemic Diseases.* Rustington, Essex, U.K.: Health Sciences Press, 1967.

Strehlow, Dr., Wighard and Gottfried Hertzka, M.D. *Hildegard of Bingen's Medicine.* Trans. Karin Anderson Strehlow. Santa Fe: Bear & Company, Inc., 1988.

Ullman, Dana, M.P.H. *The Consumer's Guide to Homeopathy.* New York: Jeremy P. Tarcher/Putnam, 1995.

Weil, Andrew, M.D. *Health and Healing.* New York: Houghton Mifflin Company, 1983.

Yiamouyiannis, Dr. John. *Fluoride the Aging Factor: How to Recognize and Avoid the Devastating Effects of Fluoride.* Delaware, OH: Health Action Press, 1986.

Zand, Janet, L.Ac., O.M.D., Rachel Walton, R.N., and Bob Roundtree, M.D. *Smart Medicine for a Healthier Child: A Practical A to Z Reference to Natural and Conventional Treatments for Infants and Children.* Garden City Park, NY: Avery Publishing Group, Inc., 1994.

INDEX

('t' indicates a table)